Quick Reference
to
Cardiovascular
Pharmacotherapy

Edited by
Judy W. M. Cheng, Pharm.D., BCPS

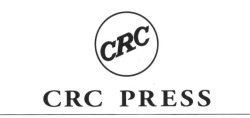

CRC PRESS

Boca Raton   London   New York   Washington, D.C.

Library of Congress Cataloging-in-Publication Data

Quick reference to cardiovascular pharmacotherapy / edited by Judy W.M. Cheng.
    p. ; cm.
Includes bibliographical references and index.
ISBN 1-58716-044-7 (alk. paper)
    1. Cardiovascular agents--Handbooks, manuals, etc. I. Cheng, Judy W. M.
[DNLM: 1. Cardiovascular Diseases--drug therapy--Handbooks. 2. Cardiovascular
Agents--administration & dosage--Handbooks. WG 39 Q67 2002]
RM345 .Q53 2002
615'.71--dc21
                                       2002067403

Visit the CRC Press Web site at www.crcpress.com

Dedications

This handbook is dedicated to all the greatest mentors
who have believed in me and inspired me in my
professional career, and most importantly, to my family,
who has provided me the best of what life can offer,
and endless support to pursue my desire.

Judy Cheng

Special thanks to my husband, David Lai, for his
unwavering support, and to my friends, mentors, and students,
without whose inspiration I would not have
been able to accomplish this work.

Angela Cheng-Lai

This work is dedicated to the many pharmacists,
physicians, nurses, and patients who have taught and inspired me
during my professional life. Above all, this is for
Joseph and Ian, who teach me daily to appreciate
what is truly important.

Sherry K. Milfred-LaForest

Dedicated to my aunt, Ita Faingerts, whose life, although abruptly halted by cancer, is a pulsating reflection of what an extraordinary woman she will always be remembered as. Her spirit, dreams, purpose continue to shape the lives of her loved ones and those touched by her kindness.

Vitalina Rozenfeld

To my mother, Geraldine, for being a continual source of support throughout this endeavor.

Cynthia Sanoski

Preface

This quick pocket reference serves as a guide for pharmacists and other health-care professionals who provide care to patients with cardiovascular diseases, and will also be useful for pharmacy trainees (fellows, residents, and students) as a collection of important evidence-based guidelines and standard of care in pharmacological management of cardiovascular diseases.

Cardiovascular diseases have always been the number one killer of Americans. Treatment of cardiovascular disorders is one of the most highly evidence-based area of medicine and pharmacy practice. This book is written based on the most updated treatment guidelines and standard of practice of different cardiovascular disorders, as well as experience of our contributors, who are clinical pharmacy specialists in cardiology or practice in environments dealing mostly with patients with cardiac disorders.

This book is not intended to be a complete text. It is a collection of important treatment algorithms and other clinical pearls that are helpful to practitioners in their day-to-day practice. The quick reference begins with management of important cardiovascular risk factors: hypertension and hyperlipidemia. Following are important pharmacotherapeutics-oriented cardiovascular disorders: stable angina, acute coronary syndrome, acute and chronic heart failure, cardiogenic shock and heart transplantation, endocarditis, and arrhythmias. In addition, we have also added two chapters tackling other important pharmacotherapeutics problems related to managing patients with cardiovascular diseases: drug-induced cardiovascular diseases and alternative pharmacotherapy used in managing cardiovascular diseases.

Perhaps the most efficient way to utilize this pocket guide is by either looking through the table of contents or by going through the index for the topic of interest. The contributors, based on their clinical experience, have incorporated information on most of the commonly encountered clinical problems in our practice. It is, however, important to realize that cardiovascular disease management is an area of constant change. Continuous research brings us new results and strategies for disease management. It is always important to keep up-to-date with the latest clinical trial results and incorporate those results into our practice appropriately.

Judy Cheng

Acknowledgment

We would like to thank the following people for providing their valuable opinions to this reference: Dr. Horatio Fung, Pharm.D., BCPS, Veterans Affairs Medical Center, Bronx, NY; Ms. Kimberly Huck, RN, ND, University Hospitals of Cleveland, Cleveland, OH; and Dr. Robert W. Stewart, M.D., University Hospitals of Cleveland, Cleveland, OH.

The Editor

Judy W.M. Cheng, Pharm.D, BCPS, is associate professor of Arnold and Marie Schwartz College of Pharmacy, Long Island University, clinical pharmacy specialist in cardiology at Mount Sinai Medical Center in New York. She is also an adjunct clinical instructor for the School of Nursing at Columbia University. Dr. Cheng received her bachelor of science degree from the University of Toronto. She then completed a clinical pharmacy residency at St. Michael's Hospital in Toronto. She received her doctor of pharmacy degree from Philadelphia College of Pharmacy and further completed a fellowship in cardiovascular pharmacotherapy at the same institution. Dr. Cheng is also a board-certified pharmacotherapy specialist with added qualification in cardiovascular pharmacotherapy.

Dr. Cheng is a member of the editorial advisory board of the *Annals of Pharmacotherapy*. She is also a member of the cardiology item writing panel for the Board Certification of Pharmaceutical Specialties Examination. Dr. Cheng is an active member of the American College of Clinical Pharmacy, the American Society of Health System Pharmacists, and the American Association of College of Pharmacy. She has also served as chair of the Cardiology Practice Relation Network of the American College of Clinical Pharmacy. Dr. Cheng's research areas of interest include cardiovascular pharmacotherapy, treatment guidelines adherence, and patient outcomes. She has published extensively in these areas.

Contributors

Judy W.M. Cheng, Pharm.D., BCPS
Associate Professor of Pharmacy Practice and Health Sciences
Long Island University
Brooklyn, New York
and
Clinical Pharmacy Specialist in Cardiology
Mount Sinai Medical Center
New York, New York

Angela Cheng-Lai, Pharm.D.
Clinical Pharmacy Manager/Adult Medicine
Montefiore Medical Center
Bronx, New York
and
Assistant Professor of Medicine
Albert Einstein College of Medicine
Bronx, New York

Sherry K. Milfred-LaForest, Pharm.D., BCPS
Clinical Pharmacist, Heart Failure and Heart Transplantion
Heart Failure Center
University Hospitals of Cleveland
Cleveland, Ohio

James Nawarskas, Pharm.D., BCPS
Assistant Professor of Clinical Pharmacy
College of Pharmacy
University of New Mexico
Albuquerque, New Mexico

Vitalina Rozenfeld, Pharm.D., BCPS
Assistant Professor of Pharmacy Practice
Long Island University
Brooklyn, New York
and
Clinical Pharmacy Specialist
Lenox Hill Hospital
New York, New York

Cynthia A. Sanoski, Pharm.D.
Assistant Professor of Clinical Pharmacy
Philadelphia College of Pharmacy
Philadelphia, Pennsylvania

Table of Contents

Chapter 2
Hyperlipidemia

Judy W.M. Cheng

Chapter 3
Pharmacologic Management of Chronic Stable Angina

James Nawarskas

Chapter 6

Chapter 7

Chapter 8
Cynthia A. Sanoski

Chapter 9
Cynthia A. Sanoski

Chapter 10
Pharmacological Management of Thromboembolic Diseases........................205
James Nawarskas

Chapter 11
Endocarditis: Prophylaxis and Treatment 223
Judy W.M. Cheng

Chapter 12
Medication-Induced Cardiovascular Side Effects..241
Cynthia A. Sanoski

1 Pharmacological Management of Hypertension

Angela Cheng-Lai

CONTENTS

Definition of Hypertension[1]

- Systolic blood pressure ≥140 mm Hg
- Diastolic blood pressure ≥90 mm Hg
- Treatment with antihypertensive medication

TABLE 1.1
Classification of Blood Pressure for Adults[a]

Category	Systolic Blood Pressure (mm Hg)		Diastolic Blood Pressure (mm Hg)
Optimal[b]	<120	and	<80
Normal	<130	and	<85
High–normal	130–139	or	85–89
Hypertension[c]			
Stage 1 (mild)	140–159	or	90–99
Stage 2 (moderate)	160–179	or	100–109
Stage 3 (severe)	≥180	or	≥110

[a] This classification of blood pressure is for individuals aged 18 years and older who are not taking antihypertensive drugs and not acutely ill. When systolic and diastolic blood pressures fall into different categories, the higher category is selected to classify the individual's blood pressure status. For example, 160/92 mm Hg is classified as stage 2 hypertension, and 174/120 mm Hg is classified as stage 3 hypertension. Isolated systolic hypertension is defined as systolic blood pressure ≥140 mm Hg and diastolic blood pressure <90 mm Hg. For example, 170/82 mm Hg is defined as stage 2 isolated systolic hypertension.

[b] Optimal blood pressure with respect to cardiovascular risk is <120/80 mm Hg. However, unusually low readings should be evaluated for clinical significance.

[c] Based on the average of two or more readings taken at each of two or more visits after an initial screening.

Source: Adapted from Joint National Committee on Prevention, Detection, Evaluation, and Treatment of High Blood Pressure. *Arch Intern Med*. 1997;157:2413. With permission.

Risk Stratification

- The presence or absence of target organ damage, additional risk factors (i.e., smoking, dyslipidemia, diabetes) as well as stages of hypertension are all important determinants of the risk for cardio-vascular disease in patients with hypertension.
- Risk stratification helps to determine the need for drug therapy.

TABLE 1.2
Risk Stratification and Treatment

Blood Pressure Category (mm Hg)	Risk Group A (No Risk Factors[a]; No TOD/CCD[b])	Risk Group B (At least One Risk Factor, Not including Diabetes; No TOD/CCD)	Risk Group C (TOD/CCD and/or Diabetes, with or without Other Risk Factors)
High-normal (130–139/85–89)	Lifestyle modification	Lifestyle modification	Drug therapy[c] and lifestyle modification
Stage 1 (140–159/90–99)	Lifestyle modification (up to 12 months)	Lifestyle modification[d] (up to 6 months)	Drug therapy and lifestyle modification
Stages 2 and 3 (≥160/≥100)	Drug therapy and lifestyle modification	Drug therapy and lifestyle modification	Drug therapy and lifestyle modification

[a] Major risk factors include smoking, dyslipidemia, diabetes mellitus, age >60 years, sex (men and postmenopausal women), and family history of cardiovascular disease in women <65 years old or in men <55 years old.

[b] TOD/CCD indicates target organ damage/clinical cardiovascular diseases, which include heart diseases (left ventricular hypertrophy, angina or prior myocardial infarction, prior coronary revascularization, and heart failure), stroke or transient ischemic attack, nephropathy, peripheral arterial disease, and retinopathy.

[c] For individuals with heart failure, renal insufficiency, or diabetes. Refer to Table 1.3 for blood pressure goals in patients with specific disease states.

[d] Clinicians should consider both drug therapy and lifestyle modification as initial treatment for patients with multiple risk factors.

Source: Adapted from Joint National Committee on Prevention, Detection, Evaluation, and Treatment of High Blood Pressure. *Arch Intern Med.* 1997;157:2413. With permission.

Objective of Prevention and Treatment of Hypertension

- To reduce the risk of cardiovascular disease and associated morbidity and mortality by the least intrusive means possible.[1]

TABLE 1.3
Blood Pressure Goals for Patients with Hypertension and Other Coexisting Diseases[a, 1-4]

Condition	Goal Blood Pressure (mm Hg)
Hypertension	<140/90
Hypertension — ambulatory blood pressure measurement	<135/85
Isolated systolic hypertension	<140/90
Diabetes	<130/80
Heart failure	<130/85
Renal insufficiency	
Without proteinuria	<130/85
With proteinuria >1 g/24 h	≤125/75

[a] Blood pressure levels obtained in the physician's office (clinic setting) except for ambulatory measurement.

Source: Adapted from Graves, JW. *Mayo Clin Proc.* 2000; 75:278. With permission.

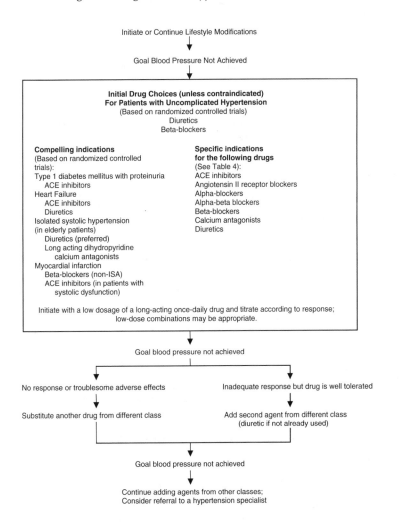

FIGURE 1.1 Algorithm for the treatment of hypertension. ACE, angiotensin-converting enzyme; ISA, intrinsic sympathomimetic activity. (From Joint National Committee on Prevention, Detection, Evaluation, and Treatment of High Blood Pressure. *Arch Intern Med.* 1997;157:2413. With permission.)

TABLE 1.4
Lifestyle Modifications for Prevention and Management of Hypertension[1,2]

Weight Reduction in Overweight Individuals
- Weight loss may be accomplished through dietary caloric restriction and increased physical activity
- Appetite suppressants, which contain sympathomimetics that can elevate blood pressure, should be avoided

Increased Aerobic Physical Activity
- Moderately intense physical activity such as 30–45 min of brisk walking, swimming, or bicycling at least three times per week (preferably once daily) is recommended

Dietary Modification
- A diet rich in fruits, vegetables, and low-fat dairy products and reduced in saturated and total fat has been shown to reduce blood pressure significantly[5]

Moderation of Dietary Sodium
- Salt intake should be limited to no more than 2.4 g of sodium or 6 g of sodium chloride per day

Potassium Intake
- An adequate intake of potassium (approximately 90 mmol/day), preferably from dietary sources such as fresh fruits and vegetables, is recommended

Calcium Intake
- An adequate intake of dietary calcium for general health is recommended

Magnesium Intake
- An adequate intake of dietary magnesium for general health is recommended

Moderation of Alcohol Intake
- Alcohol consumption should be limited to no more than 1 oz of ethanol (e.g., 24 oz of beer, 10 oz of wine, or 2 oz of 100-proof whiskey) per day for most men and 0.5 oz of ethanol per day for women and lighter-weight individuals

Smoking Avoidance/Cessation
- Avoidance of tobacco is essential for the prevention of cardiovascular disease

TABLE 1.5
Use of Antihypertensive Drug Therapy in Patients with Comorbid Conditions

Indication	Drug Therapy
Compelling Indications Unless Contraindicated	
Diabetes mellitus (type 1) with or without proteinuria	ACE inhibitors
Heart failure	ACE inhibitors, diuretics, beta-blockers
Isolated systolic hypertension (older patients)	Diuretics (preferred), calcium antagonists (long-acting dihydropyridine)
Myocardial infarction	Beta-blockers (non-ISA), ACE inhibitors
May Have Favorable Effects on Comorbid Conditions	
Angina	Beta-blockers, calcium antagonists (long-acting)
Atrial tachycardia and fibrillation	Beta-blockers, calcium antagonists (non-dihydropyridine)
Cyclosporine-induced hypertension	Calcium antagonists
Diabetes mellitus (types 1 and 2) without proteinuria	ACE inhibitors (preferred), calcium antagonists
Diabetes mellitus (type 2)	Diuretics (low-dose)
Dyslipidemia	Alpha-blockers
Essential tremor	Beta-blockers (noncardioselective)
Heart failure	Beta-blockers, angiotensin II receptor blockers, spironolactone
Hyperthyroidism	Beta-blockers
Migraine headache	Beta-blockers (noncardioselective), calcium antagonists (nondihydropyridine)
Myocardial infarction	Diltiazem, verapamil
Osteoporosis	Thiazides
Preoperative hypertension	Beta-blockers
Prostatism (benign prostatic hyperplasia)	Alpha-blockers
Renal insufficiency (caution in renovascular hypertension and creatinine concentration ≥3 mg/dl)	ACE inhibitors

TABLE 1.5 (CONTINUED)
Use of Antihypertensive Drug Therapy in Patients with Comorbid Conditions

Indication	Drug Therapy
May Have Unfavorable Effects on Comorbid Conditions[a]	
Bronchospastic disease	Beta-blockers[b]
Depression	Beta-blockers, central alpha-agonists, reserpine[b]
Diabetes mellitus (types 1 and 2)	Beta-blockers, diuretics (high-dose)
Dyslipidemia	Beta-blockers (non-ISA), diuretics (high-dose)
Gout	Diuretics
Heart block (second or third degree)	Beta-blockers[b], diltiazem[b], verapamil[b]
Heart failure	Calcium antagonists (except amlodipine and felodipine)
Liver disease	Labetalol, methyldopa[b]
Peripheral vascular disease	Beta-blockers
Pregnancy	ACE inhibitors[b], angiotensin II receptor blockers[b]
Renal insufficiency	Potassium-sparing agents
Renovascular disease	ACE inhibitors, angiotensin II receptor blockers

[a] These drugs may be used with special monitoring unless contraindicated.

[b] Contraindicated.

ACE, angiotensin-converting enzyme; ISA, intrinsic sympathomimetic activity.

Source: Adapted from Joint National Committee on Prevention, Detection, Evaluation, and Treatment of High Blood Pressure. *Arch Intern Med*. 1997;157:2413. With permission.

TABLE 1.6
Dosage and Therapeutic Considerations for Oral Antihypertensive Medications[a] [1,6-11]

Drug	Initial Dose[b]	Maximum Dose	Comments
Alpha-Adrenergic Blockers			
Doxazosin	1 mg po qd	16 mg/day (qd or bid dosing)	This class of drugs is generally not used as first-line agents in hypertension. A recent randomized trial found an increased incidence of cardiovascular events, particularly congestive heart failure, in high-risk with hypertensive patients treated with doxazosin compared to those treated with chlorthalidone.[7] Postural hypotension is a possible adverse effect. Careful blood pressure monitoring for hypotension and orthostasis is recommended, especially for elderly patients.
Prazosin	1 mg po bid or tid	20 mg/day (bid or tid dosing)	
Terazosin	1 mg po hs	20 mg/day (qd or bid dosing)	
Alpha₂-Adrenergic Agonists			
Clonidine	0.05–0.1 mg po bid	2.4 mg/day (bid or tid dosing)	These agents are generally not used as initial monotherapy for hypertension due to their unfavorable side effect profiles. Some possible adverse effects are hypotension, sedation, and dry mouth. Treatment with this group of agents should not be discontinued abruptly. Methyldopa has been recommended for women whose hypertension is first diagnosed during pregnancy.[1]
Guanabenz	4 mg po bid	16 mg po bid	
Guanfacine	1 mg po hs	3 mg po qd	
Methyldopa	250 mg po bid or tid	3000 mg/day (bid or tid dosing)	

TABLE 1.6 (CONTINUED)
Dosage and Therapeutic Considerations for Oral Antihypertensive Medications[a] [1,6-11]

Drug	Initial Dose[b]	Maximum Dose	Comments
Angiotensin-Converting Enzyme Inhibitors			
Benazepril	10 mg po qd	80 mg/day (qd or bid dosing)	These agents are particularly beneficial in patients with
Captopril[c]	12.5 mg po bid or tid	50 mg po tid	hypertension-related processes such as heart failure from systolic
Enalapril	5 mg po qd	20 mg po bid	dysfunction and nephropathy.[1]
Fosinopril	10 mg po qd	40 mg/day (qd or bid dosing)	ACE inhibitors are also useful after myocardial infarction to prevent
Lisinopril	10 mg po qd	40 mg po qd	subsequent heart failure and
Moexipril[c]	7.5 mg po qd	30 mg/day (qd or bid dosing)	mortality.[1] There appears to be little difference among the ACE
Perindopril	4 mg po qd	16 mg/day	inhibitors in antihypertensive
Quinapril	10 mg po qd	80 mg/day (qd or bid dosing)	efficacy. When administered at effective doses, studies comparing
Ramipril	2.5 mg po qd	20 mg/day (qd or bid dosing)	antihypertensive efficacy among the different agents do not
Trandolapril	1 mg po qd	8 mg/day (qd or bid dosing)	consistently show greater efficacy of one agent vs. another.[8] The most common adverse effect encountered with ACE inhibitors is cough. Other possible side effects include headache, dizziness, rash, increased BUN or serum creatinine, hyperkalemia, and angioedema (rare).

TABLE 1.6 (CONTINUED)
Dosage and Therapeutic Considerations for Oral Antihypertensive Medications[a] [1,6-11]

Drug	Initial Dose[b]	Maximum Dose	Comments
Angiotensin-II Receptor Blockers			
Candesartan	16 mg po qd	32 mg po qd	These agents produce
Eprosartan	600 mg po qd	800 mg/day (qd or bid dosing)	hemodynamic effects similar to those of ACE inhibitors while
Irbesartan	150 mg po qd	300 mg po qd	avoiding the most common
Losartan	50 mg po qd	100 mg/day (qd or bid dosing)	adverse effect, dry cough.[1] However, in the absence of data
Telmisartan	40 mg po qd	80 mg po qd	demonstrating equal long-term
Valsartan	80 mg po qd	320 mg po qd	protection in patients with hypertension-related processes such as heart failure from systolic dysfunction and nephropathy, angiotensin II receptor blockers should be used primarily in patients in whom ACE inhibitors are indicated but who are unable to tolerate them.[1,9] Possible adverse effects include headache, dizziness, upper respiratory tract infection, increased BUN or serum creatinine, hyperkalemia, and angioedema (rare).

TABLE 1.6 (CONTINUED)
Dosage and Therapeutic Considerations for Oral Antihypertensive Medications[a] [1,6-11]

Drug	Initial Dose[b]	Maximum Dose	Comments
Beta-Adrenergic Blockers			
Nonselective Beta-Adrenergic Blockers without ISA			
Nadolol	20–40 mg po qd	320 mg po qd	When there are no indications for another type of drug, initial antihypertensive therapy with a beta-blocker or diuretic is recommended because numerous randomized controlled trials have shown a reduction in morbidity and mortality with these agents.[1] The use of beta-blockers without ISA after myocardial infarction has been shown to reduce the risk for subsequent myocardial infarction or sudden cardiac death.[1] Because beta-blockers and alpha-beta-blockers may exacerbate asthma, these agents should be avoided in patients with asthma except in special circumstances.[1] Agents with beta$_1$ selectivity in low to moderate doses may be safer than nonselective agents in patients with reactive airways disease. Possible adverse effects of beta-blockers include bronchospasm, bradycardia, heart failure, postural hypotension, fatigue, impaired peripheral circulation, hypertriglyceridemia (except agents with ISA), and male
Propranolol (immediate-release)	40 mg po bid	640 mg/day (bid or tid dosing)	
Propranolol (extended-release)	80 mg po qd	640 mg/day	
Timolol	10 mg po bid	30 mg po bid	
Beta$_1$ Selective Beta-Adrenergic Blockers without ISA			
Atenolol	50 mg po qd	100 mg/day (qd or bid dosing)	
Betaxolol	10 mg po qd	20–40 mg po qd	
Bisoprolol	2.5–5 mg po qd	20 mg po qd	
Metoprolol (immediate-release)	50 mg po bid	450 mg/day (in divided doses)	
Metoprolol (extended-release)	100 mg po qd	450 mg/day	
Beta-Adrenergic Blockers with ISA			
Acebutolol	200 mg po qd	600 mg po bid	
Carteolol	2.5 mg po qd	10 mg po qd	
Penbutolol	20 mg po qd	20 mg po qd	
Pindolol	5 mg po bid	30 mg po bid	

TABLE 1.6 (CONTINUED)
Dosage and Therapeutic Considerations for Oral Antihypertensive Medications[a] [1,6-11]

Drug	Initial Dose[b]	Maximum Dose	Comments
Combined Alpha- and Beta-Blockers			impotence. In addition, beta-blockers may mask insulin-induced hypoglycemia.
Carvedilol	6.25 mg po bid	25 mg po bid	
Labetalol	100 mg po bid	1200–2400 mg/day (bid or tid dosing)	

Calcium Antagonists

Drug	Initial Dose	Maximum Dose	Comments
Amlodipine	5 mg po qd	10 mg po qd	This group of agents may be particularly useful in patients with hypertension and angina pectoris.[1] In addition, calcium antagonists are recommended for elderly patients with systolic hypertension and for black patients.[10] Calcium antagonists may be classified based on their chemical structures. Verapamil is a phenylalkylamine and a first-generation calcium antagonist. Diltiazem is a benzothiazepine as well as a first-generation calcium antagonist. The largest group of calcium antagonists is the dihydropyridines, which include the first-generation agents nifedipine and nicardipine, the second-generation agents felodipine ER, isradipine, nicardipine SR, nisoldipine, and nimodipine, and the third-generation agent amlodipine.[11]
Diltiazem (Cardizem SR)	60 mg po bid	180 mg po bid	
Diltiazem (Cardizem CD)	120 mg po qd	360 mg po qd	
Felodipine (extended-release)	5 mg po qd	10 mg po qd	
Isradipine (DynaCirc)	2.5 mg po bid	10 mg po bid	
Isradipine (DynaCirc CR)	5 mg po qd	20 mg po qd	
Nicardipine (Cardene)	20 mg po tid	40 mg po tid	
Nicardipine[d] (Cardene SR)	30 mg po bid	60 mg po bid	
Nifedipine[e] (Adalat CC)	30 mg po qd	90 mg po qd	
Nifedipine[e] (Procardia XL)	30–60 mg po qd	120 mg po qd	
Nisoldipine[f]	20 mg po qd	60 mg po qd	
Verapamil (immediate-release)	80 mg po tid	160 mg po tid	

TABLE 1.6 (CONTINUED)
Dosage and Therapeutic Considerations for Oral Antihypertensive Medications[a] [1,6-11]

Drug	Initial Dose[b]	Maximum Dose	Comments
Verapamil (sustained-release)	120 mg po qd	480 mg/day (qd or bid dosing)	Possible adverse effects from nondihydropyridine calcium antagonists include bradycardia, conduction defects, worsening of systolic dysfunction, headache, dizziness, peripheral edema, and constipation (verapamil). Possible adverse effects from dihydropyridines include peripheral edema, palpitations, tachycardia, headache, dizziness, asthenia, flushing, and gingival hyperplasia (rare).
Verapamil (extended-release, controlled onset)	180–200 mg po hs	400–540 mg po hs	

Diuretics

Thiazide Diuretics

Drug	Initial Dose[b]	Maximum Dose	Comments
Chlorthalidone[g] (Hygroton)	25 mg po qd	100 mg po qd	Diuretics have been proved in controlled clinical trials to reduce hypertensive morbidity and mortality in African Americans as well as in whites; thus, diuretics should be the agent of first choice for the management of hypertension unless contraindicated.[1] Diuretics are also particularly recommended for the treatment of elderly patients with systolic hypertension and of black patients.[10] Thiazide diuretics are not effective in patients with advanced renal insufficiency (serum creatinine ≥2.5 mg/dl), and
Chlorthalidone[g] (Thalitone)	15 mg po qd	50 mg po qd	
Hydrochloro-thiazide	12.5–25 mg po qd	50 mg po qd	
Indapamide	1.25 mg po qd	5 mg po qd	
Metolazone (Mykrox)	0.5 mg po qd	1 mg po qd	
Metolazone (Zaroxolyn)	2.5 mg po qd	10 mg po qd	

Loop Diuretics

Furosemide	40 mg po bid	240 mg/day (bid or tid dosing)	
Torsemide	5 mg po qd	10 mg po qd	

TABLE 1.6 (CONTINUED)
Dosage and Therapeutic Considerations for Oral Antihypertensive Medications[a] [1,6-11]

Drug	Initial Dose[b]	Maximum Dose	Comments
Potassium-Sparing Diuretics			loop diuretics are needed (often at
Amiloride	5 mg po qd	10 mg po qd	relatively large doses). In patients
Spironolactone	25 mg po qd	100 mg/day (qd or bid dosing)	who are resistant to a loop diuretic alone, combining a loop diuretic
Triamterene	50 mg po qd	100 mg po qd	with a thiazide diuretic such as

metolazone may prove to be effective.[1] Potassium-sparing diuretics such as spironolactone and triamterene are often used in combination with a thiazide diuretic for the management of hypertension; these agents should be avoided in patients with renal impairment. In high doses, thiazide diuretics and loop diuretics can induce at least short-term elevations in total plasma cholesterol, triglyceride, and low-density lipoprotein cholesterol concentration.[1] All diuretics can increase serum uric acid concentrations but rarely induce acute gout. Diuretics should be avoided if possible in patients with gout.[1] Other possible adverse effects of diuretics include hypotension, dizziness, ototoxicity (loop diuretics), volume and electrolyte depletion, hyperglycemia, hyperkalemia (potassium-sparing diuretics), and gynecomastia (spironolactone).

TABLE 1.6 (CONTINUED)
Dosage and Therapeutic Considerations for Oral Antihypertensive Medications[a] [1,6-11]

Drug	Initial Dose[b]	Maximum Dose	Comments
Neuronal and Ganglionic Blockers			
Guanadrel	5 mg po bid	75 mg/day (bid, tid, or qid dosing)	These agents are usually not used as initial monotherapy for hypertension due to their
Guanethidine	10 mg po qd	50 mg po qd	unfavorable side effect profiles.
Reserpine[h]	0.5 mg po qd for 1 or 2 weeks (if given as mono-therapy)[i]	0.1–0.25 mg po qd (usual maintenance dose)	Possible adverse effects include orthostatic hypotension, diarrhea, nasal congestion, sedation, depression, and activation of peptic ulcer (reserpine).
Vasodilators			
Hydralazine	10 mg po qid	300 mg/day (bid dosing may be adequate)	These agents are usually not used as initial monotherapy for hypertension due to their
Minoxidil	5 mg po qd	100 mg/day (qd or bid dosing)	unfavorable side effect profiles. Hydralazine and minoxidil often induce reflex sympathetic stimulation of the cardiovascular system and fluid retention.[1] Other possible adverse effects include lupus-like syndrome (hydralazine) and hirsutism (minoxidil).

[a] Medications are listed in alphabetical order by category.

[b] The following are usual initial doses in adult patients. Patients with renal or hepatic impairment may require lower initial doses.

[c] Advise patients to take captopril and moexipril 1 h before meals.

TABLE 1.6 (CONTINUED)
Dosage and Therapeutic Considerations for Oral Antihypertensive Medications[a] [1,6-11]

[d] The total daily dose of immediate-release nicardipine may not be a useful guide in determining the effective dose of the sustained release form start titrate patients currently receiving the immediate-release form with the sustained release form at their current daily dose of immediate-release, then reexamine to evaluate the adequacy of blood pressure control.

[e] Immediate-release nifedipine has precipitated ischemic events and, in large doses, may increase coronary mortality in patients who have had a myocardial infarction.[1] Manufacturer's labeling states that the immediate-release formulation should not be used for hypertension, hypertensive crisis, acute myocardial infarction, and some forms of unstable angina and chronic stable angina.

[f] Administration of nisoldipine with a high-fat meal can lead to excessive peak drug concentration and should be avoided. In addition, grapefruit products should be avoided before and after dosing.

[g] Dosages >25 mg/day (Thalitone, 15 mg/day) are likely to potentiate potassium loss, but provide no further benefit in sodium excretion or blood pressure reduction.

[h] Reserpine should be taken with meals to avoid gastric irritation.

[i] Reserpine should be initiated at a lower dose of 0.05 mg daily in elderly individuals; dosage may be increased by 0.05 mg/day every week as needed and tolerated.

ISA = intrinsic sympathomimetic activity.

TABLE 1.7
Pharmacologic Properties of Oral Antihypertensive Medications

Drug	Onset of Action	Peak Effect	Duration of Action	Half-Life[a]	Primary Route(s) of Elimination
Alpha-Adrenergic Blockers					
Doxazosin	1–2 h	4–8 h	24 h	19–22 h	Hepatic
Prazosin	<2 h[b]	2–4 h[c]	<24 h	2–4 h	Hepatic
Terazosin	<1 h	3–4 h	>24 h	12 h	Hepatic
Alpha$_2$-Adrenergic Agonists					
Clonidine	30–60 min	2–4 h	8–12 h	12–16 h	Hepatic/renal
Guanabenz	1 h	2–4 h	≥10–12 h	12–14 h	Hepatic
Guanfacine	2 h	6 h	≥24 h	10–30 h	Hepatic/renal
Methyldopa	3–6 h	6–9 h	24–48 h	90–127 min	Hepatic
Angiotensin-Converting Enzyme Inhibitors					
Benazepril	1 h	2–6 h	≤24 h	10–11 h (benazeprilat)	Renal
Captopril	15–60 min	60–90 min	6–12 h	2 h	Renal
Enalapril	≈1 h	4–6 h	≤24 h	11 h (enalaprilat)	Renal
Fosinopril	1 h	2–7 h	24 h	12 h (fosinoprilat)	Hepatic/renal
Lisinopril	1 h	6 h	24 h	12 h	Renal
Moexipril	1 h	3–6 h	≤24 h	12 h (moexiprilat)	Hepatic/renal
Perindopril	≈1 h	3–7 h	≈24 h	3–10 h[d]	Renal
Quinapril	1 h	2–4 h	≤24 h	≈3 h (quinaprilat)	Renal
Ramipril	1–2 h	3–6 h	≤24 h	13–17 h (ramiprilat)	Renal
Trandolapril	4 h	6 h	≥24 h	10 h (trandolaprilat)	Hepatic/renal
Angiotensin-II Receptor Blockers					
Candesartan	2–4 h	6–8 h	≥24 h	≈9 h	Hepatic/renal

TABLE 1.7 (CONTINUED)
Pharmacologic Properties of Oral Antihypertensive Medications

Drug	Onset of Action	Peak Effect	Duration of Action	Half-Life[a]	Primary Route(s) of Elimination
Eprosartan	1–2 h	3 h	≤24 h	5–9 h	Hepatic/biliary
Irbesartan	2 h	3–6 h	24 h	11–15 h	Hepatic
Losartan	2–3 h	6 h	24 h	2 h (parent compound)[e]	Hepatic
Telmisartan	3 h	3–9 h	≥24 h	≈24 h	Hepatic/biliary
Valsartan	2 h	4–6 h	≈24 h	≈6 h	Hepatic

Beta-Adrenergic Blockers

Nonselective Beta-Adrenergic Blockers without ISA

Drug	Onset of Action	Peak Effect	Duration of Action	Half-Life[a]	Primary Route(s) of Elimination
Nadolol	<2 h	2–4 hours	>24 h	10–24 h	Renal
Propranolol (immediate-release)	1–2 h[f]	60–90 min	≈6 h	3–6 h	Hepatic
Propranolol (extended-release)	1–2 h[f]	6 h	≤24 h	3–6 h	Hepatic
Timolol	30 min	1–2 h	12–24 h	4 h	Hepatic

Beta₁ Selective Beta-Adrenergic Blockers without ISA

Drug	Onset of Action	Peak Effect	Duration of Action	Half-Life[a]	Primary Route(s) of Elimination
Atenolol	≈1 h	2–4 h[g]	≈24 h	6–7 h	Renal
Betaxolol	2–3 h	3–4 h	>24 h	14–22 h	Hepatic
Bisoprolol	1–2 h	2–4 h[h]	≈24 h	9–12 h	Hepatic/renal
Metoprolol (immediate-release)	<1 h	1–2 h	≈12 h	3–7 h	Hepatic
Metoprolol (extended-release)	≈1 h	>7 h	≥24 h	3–7 h	Hepatic

Beta-Adrenergic Blockers with ISA

Drug	Onset of Action	Peak Effect	Duration of Action	Half-Life[a]	Primary Route(s) of Elimination
Acebutolol	1–2 h	3–8 h	≈24 h	3–4 h[i]	Hepatic/biliary
Carteolol	1–3 h	6 h	>24 h	6 h[j]	Renal

TABLE 1.7 (CONTINUED)
Pharmacologic Properties of Oral Antihypertensive Medications

Drug	Onset of Action	Peak Effect	Duration of Action	Half-Life[a]	Primary Route(s) of Elimination
Penbutolol	<1 h	2–3 h	>20 h	5 h	Hepatic
Pindolol	<3 h	3–4 h[k]	24 h	3–4 h	Hepatic/renal
Combined Alpha- and Beta-Blockers					
Carvedilol	1 h	4–7 h	12–24 h	7–10 h	Hepatic/biliary
Labetalol	1–2 h	2–4 h	8–24 h	6–8 h	Hepatic
Calcium Antagonists					
Amlodipine	30–50 min[l]	6–12 h	24 h	30–50 h	Hepatic
Diltiazem (Cardizem SR)	30–60 min	3–6 h	≈12 h	5–7 h	Hepatic
Diltiazem (Cardizem CD)	30–60 min	≈10 h[m]	24 h	5–7 h	Hepatic
Felodipine (extended-release)	2–5 h	4–8 h	16–24 h	11–16 h	Hepatic
Isradipine (DynaCirc)	1 h	2–3 h	12 h	8 h	Hepatic
Isradipine (DynaCirc CR)	2 h	8–10 h	24 h	8 h	Hepatic
Nicardipine (Cardene)	20 min	≈2 h	8 h	8 h	Hepatic
Nicardipine (Cardene SR)	<1 h	4 h	12 h	8 h	Hepatic
Nifedipine (Adalat CC)	<1 h	2–6 h	≤24 h	2–5 h	Hepatic
Nifedipine (Procardia XL)	<1 h	2–6 h	≤24 h	2–5 h	Hepatic
Nisoldipine (extended-release)	ND	ND	24 h	7–12 h	Hepatic

TABLE 1.7 (CONTINUED)
Pharmacologic Properties of Oral Antihypertensive Medications

Drug	Onset of Action	Peak Effect	Duration of Action	Half-Life[a]	Primary Route(s) of Elimination
Verapamil (immediate-release)	≤1 h	2 h	8 h	4–12 h	Hepatic
Verapamil (extended-release, controlled onset)	≈5 h	≈12 h	24 h	4–12 h	Hepatic

Diuretics

Thiazide Diuretics

Chlorthalidone	2–3 h	2–6 h	≤72 h	40–60 h	Renal
Hydrochloro-thiazide	2 h[n]	3-6 h	6–12 h	6–15 h	Renal
Indapamide	1–2 h[o]	≈2 h[o]	≤36 h	≥14 h	Hepatic
Metolazone	≤1 h	1–2 h[p]	12–24 h	8–14 h	Renal

Loop Diuretics

Furosemide	30–60 min[q]	1–2 h[q]	6–8 h	0.5–2 h	Renal
Torsemide	<1 h[r]	1–2 h[r]	8–12 h	3.5 h	Hepatic

Potassium-Sparing Diuretics

Amiloride	2 h[s]	6–10 h[s]	24 h	6–9 h	Renal
Spironolactone	2 h[t]	6–8 h[t]	48–72 h	1–2 h (parent drug)[u]	Hepatic/biliary/renal
Triamterene	2–4 h[v]	Several days[v]	7–9 h	1.5–2.5 h	Hepatic/renal

Neuronal and Ganglionic Blockers

Guanadrel	2 h	4–6 h	9 h (4–14 h)	10 h	Hepatic/renal

TABLE 1.7 (CONTINUED)
Pharmacologic Properties of Oral Antihypertensive Medications

Drug	Onset of Action	Peak Effect	Duration of Action	Half-Life[a]	Primary Route(s) of Elimination
Guanethidine	0.5–2 h	2–16 days	24–48 h	36 h (alpha); 96–192 h (beta)	Hepatic/renal
Reserpine	Several days	Days to weeks	1–6 weeks	4.5 h (initial); 45–168 h (terminal)	Hepatic/fecal
Vasodilators					
Hydralazine	45 min	1 h	6–12 h	3–7 h	Hepatic
Minoxidil	30 min	4–8 h	≤100 h	4.2 h	Hepatic

[a] Half-life may increase significantly in patients with renal or hepatic impairment.

[b] The first antihypertensive response to prazosin occurs within 2 weeks of drug initiation.

[c] The peak antihypertensive response to prazosin occurs at 4–8 weeks after initiation of therapy.

[d] Apparent plasma half-life of perindoprilat; terminal elimination half-life of perindoprilat is 30–120 h.

[e] Active metabolite of losartan, E3174, has a half-life of approximately 6–9 hours.

[f] The time listed here is the time to onset of beta blockade effect; the first antihypertensive response to propranolol may occur at 2–3 weeks after initiation of therapy.

[g] The peak antihypertensive response to atenolol occurs at 3–14 days after initiation of therapy.

[h] The peak antihypertensive response to bisoprolol occurs within 2–6 weeks after initiation of therapy.

[i] Active metabolite of acebutolol, diacetolol, has a half-life of 8–13 h.

[j] Active metabolite of carteolol, 8-hydroxycarteolol, has a half-life of 8–12 h.

[k] The peak antihypertensive response to pindolol occurs within 1–2 weeks after initiation of therapy.

[l] The first antihypertensive response to amlodipine occurs at 24–96 h after initiation of therapy.

[m] The peak antihypertensive response to Cardizem CD® may not be apparent for up to 14 days after initiation of therapy.

[n] The time listed here is the time to onset of diuresis; the first antihypertensive response to hydrochlorothiazide may occur at 3–4 days after initiation of therapy.

TABLE 1.7 (CONTINUED)
Pharmacologic Properties of Oral Antihypertensive Medications

[o] The time listed here is the time to effect on diuresis. The first antihypertensive response to indapamide may occur within 1 week after initiation of therapy; the peak antihypertensive response to indapamide may occur within 8–12 weeks after initiation of therapy.

[p] The peak antihypertensive response to metolazone may occur within 2 weeks after initiation of therapy.

[q] The time listed here is the time to effect on diuresis; the peak antihypertensive response to furosemide may occur several days after initiation of therapy.

[r] The time listed here is the time to effect on diuresis. The first antihypertensive response to torsemide may occur within 1 week after initiation of therapy; the peak antihypertensive response to torsemide may occur at 8–12 weeks after initiation of therapy.

[s] The time listed here is the time to effect on diuresis and electrolyte excretion.

[t] The time listed here is the time to effect on aldosterone antagonism; the peak diuresis response to spironolactone may occur within 2 weeks after initiation of therapy.

[u] Active metabolite of spironolactone, canrenone, has a half-life of 13–24 h.

[v] The time listed here is the time to effect on diuresis; the peak antihypertensive response to triamterene may occur at 2–3 months after initiation of therapy.

ND = no data.

TABLE 1.8
Follow-Up Plans[3,12-15]

Medications Issues to Be Discussed with Patients

Goals and expected outcomes of treatment

Dosing of drugs

Possible side effects

    Report of adverse effects from medications to health care provider when they occur

    Medication regimen should be modified to avoid/decrease the occurrence of side
      effects when necessary

Coping mechanisms for complicated medical regimens

    Utilization of time charts and pillboxes

    Assistance from family members or visiting nurses

Importance of compliance with treatment care plan

Cost of treatment

Lifestyle Modification to Be Discussed with Patients

Increased physical activity

Modification of diet and sodium intake (see Table 1.3)

Avoidance of foods/drugs that can increase blood pressure[12]

    Examples include adrenal steroids, alcohol, amphetamines, caffeine, cocaine,
      licorice, nasal decongestants, appetite suppressants, and nonsteroidal anti-
      inflammatory drugs

Enhancement of Patient Compliance to Medical Regimen

Patient education[12-14]

    Risk factors clearly stated and repeatedly emphasized

    Involvement of patient in decision making regarding therapy

    Measurement of blood pressure at home by patient or patient's family members

    Participation in support groups

Effective blood pressure control[1,3,13]

    Medication dosage titration should be done cautiously but expeditiously to achieve
      blood pressure control

    Unsuccessful therapy should be replaced with alternative treatment

    Pathophysiology of resistant hypertension should be characterized to allow for
      effective modification of therapy

    Patients with plasma volume expansion should receive intensified diuretic therapy

Simplicity of medication regimen[3,13,15]

    Utilization of long-acting agents that can be dosed once daily

TABLE 1.8 (CONTINUED)
Follow-Up Plans[3,12-15]

Utilization of combination therapy

Combination therapy offers synergy of action from more than one medication while decreasing the number of pills required per day

Lower incidence of adverse effects may be observed with combination therapy because doses of each component are usually lower than those required for monotherapy

Examples of various combinations are diuretics plus ACE inhibitors, diuretics plus angiotensin II blockers, diuretics plus beta-blockers, and calcium antagonists with ACE inhibitors

Safety and tolerance of medication regimen[13]

Treatment should have little or no interference with patient's usual lifestyle

Alternative medications should be considered when adverse effects occur

Cost-effectiveness of medication regimen[14]

Medication(s) dosage and dosing schedule may be selected to minimize patients' medication cost

Substitution with generic medications may be provided when appropriate

Frequent visits to health care provider[3]

Frequent patient visits (at least once every 3 months) to health care provider allow proper adjustment of antihypertensive regimen that is essential for the achievement of goal blood pressure

Team approach to hypertension management[3]

Teams, which consist of the patient, physician, nurse educator, pharmacist, and dietitian, can optimize blood pressure control

Consideration of Other Factors Which Affect Blood Pressure Control

Concomitant medications that can increase blood pressure[12]

Examples include adrenal steroids, amphetamines, cyclosporine, disulfiram, erythropoietin, monoamine oxidase inhibitors (combined with foods containing tyramine or with amphetamine), medications containing sodium (e.g., antacids or certain parenteral antibiotics), nonsteroidal anti-inflammatory drugs, oral contraceptives, and sympathomimetic agents

Coexisting conditions[12]

Conditions that can either increase blood pressure or interfere with its management include anxiety disorders (hyperventilation or panic attacks), delirium (with agitation and autonomic excess), hyperinsulinism with insulin resistance, obesity, pain (acute or chronic), pregnancy, and sleep apnea

TABLE 1.8 (CONTINUED)
Follow-Up Plans[3,12-15]

Disease progression

Inaccurate blood pressure measurement[12]

    Blood pressure measurements should be repeated under good conditions and with proper technique

Secondary hypertension[3,12]

    Examples of underlying disorders include renal artery stenosis, primary aldosteronism, and pheochromocytoma

Suboptimal treatment[12]

    Medication regimens should be reviewed by clinicians regularly to ensure optimal blood pressure control

White coat hypertension[12]

    Blood pressure measurements should be repeated under ambulatory settings

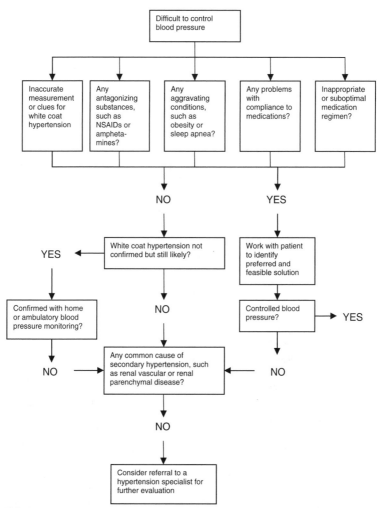

FIGURE 1.2 Evaluation and management of resistant hypertension. Resistant hypertension is defined as failure to reduce blood pressure to <140/90 mm Hg in patients who are complying with adequate triple drug regimens in appropriate dosages.[12] Although the recommendations have been presented sequentially, clinicians may consider many of the treatment options simultaneously and use their own judgment regarding the appropriate order of queries[12] NSAIDS = nonsteroidal anti-inflammatory drugs. (Adapted from O'Rorke JE, Richardson WS. *Br Med J*. 2001;322:1229.

TABLE 1.9
Hypertensive Urgency and Emergency [1,16-18]

	Hypertensive Emergency	Hypertensive Urgency
Definition	A sudden increase in systolic and diastolic blood pressure associated with end-organ damage[16]	Severely elevated blood pressure without acute end-organ damage[16]
Therapeutic approach	Immediate control of blood pressure is required to terminate ongoing end-organ damage, but not to return blood pressure to normal levels.[16,17] The initial goal of therapy is to reduce mean arterial blood pressure by no more than 20–25% within a period of minutes to 2 h depending on the clinical situation.[1,18] Alternatively, a reduction in diastolic blood pressure to 100–110 mm Hg over minutes to hours may serve as an initial goal.[18] More rapid reduction in blood pressure should be avoided because excessive falls in pressure can precipitate renal, cerebral, or coronary ischemia.[1,18]	Blood pressure may be lowered gradually over a period of 24 to 48 h.[16,17]
	The elevated blood pressure should be treated in an intensive care unit; an arterial line should be placed for accurate monitoring of blood pressure.[16,18]	Following a period of monitoring in the hospital or clinic setting, the patient can safely be discharged with close outpatient follow-up and adjustment of therapy.[18]
	Intravenous administration of antihypertensive drugs is generally preferred (see Table 1.10).	Oral medications with relatively fast onset of action may be used. The choices include loop diuretics, beta-blockers, ACE inhibitors, alpha$_2$-agonists, or calcium antagonists (see Table 1.7).[1]

ACE = angiotensin-converting enzyme.

TABLE 1.10
Parenteral Drugs for the Management of Hypertensive Emergencies[1,6,16-18]

Drug	Dose	Onset of Action	Duration of Action	Adverse Effects
Vasodilators				
Diazoxide	1–3 mg/kg (up to 150 mg) IV bolus, q 5–15 min; repeat q 4–24 h as needed	1–4 min	2–12 h	Hypotension, dizziness, flushing, tachycardia, nausea, vomiting, hyperglycemia, aggravation of angina, fluid retention
Enalaprilat	1.25–5 mg q 6 h IV[a]	15 min	6 h	Precipitous fall in blood pressure in high-renin states, variable response
Fenoldopam mesylate	0.1–1.6 µg/kg/min as IV infusion	≈5 min	≈1 h	Hypotension, reflex tachycardia (dose-related), headache, dizziness, nausea, flushing, hypokalemia, increased intraocular pressure[b]
Hydralazine hydrochloride	10–20 mg IV, 10–50 mg IM	10–20 min	3–8 h	Tachycardia, flushing, headache, vomiting, aggravation of angina
Nicardipine hydrochloride	5–15 mg/h as IV infusion	5–20 min	1–4 h	Reflex tachycardia, headache, dizziness, lightheadedness, flushing, local phlebitis

TABLE 1.10 (CONTINUED)
Parenteral Drugs for the Management of Hypertensive Emergencies[1,6,16-18]

Drug	Dose	Onset of Action	Duration of Action	Adverse Effects
Nitroglycerin	5–100 µg/min as IV infusion	Almost immediate	3–5 min	Hypotension, headache, dizziness, lightheadedness, vomiting, methemoglobinemia (usually with overdose), tolerance with prolonged use
Sodium nitroprusside	0.25–10 µg/kg/min as IV infusion (maximal dose for 10 min only)	Almost immediate	1-10 min after infusion is discontinued	Hypotension, nausea, vomiting, muscle twitching, cyanide or thiocyanate toxicity, increased intracranial pressure
Trimethaphan[c]	0.5–1 mg/min as IV infusion; increased by 0.5 mg/min as tolerated and needed; usual maintenance infusion rate is 1–5 mg/min	Almost immediate	10–15 min	Orthostatic hypotension, tachycardia, nausea, urinary retention, paralytic ileus, tachyphylaxis
Adrenergic inhibitors				
Esmolol hydrochloride	250–500 µg/kg/min for 1 min, then 50–100 µg/kg/min for 4 min; may repeat sequence	1–2 min	10–20 min	Hypotension, dizziness, bradycardia or heart block, nausea

TABLE 1.10 (CONTINUED)
Parenteral Drugs for the Management of Hypertensive Emergencies[1,6,16-18]

Drug	Dose	Onset of Action	Duration of Action	Adverse Effects
Labetalol hydrochloride	20–80 mg IV bolus, repeat every 10 min as needed (maximum total dose, 300 mg); or 2 mg/min IV infusion	2–10 min	2–4 h	Orthostatic hypotension, bradycardia, heart block, dizziness, bronchospasm, nausea, scalp tingling
Phentolamine	5–15 mg IV	Almost immediate	10–30 min	Hypotension, tachycardia, dizziness, flushing, nausea, aggravation of angina

[a] Enalaprilat may be given as intravenous injection of 1.25 mg over 5 min every 6 h, titrated by increments of 1.25 mg at 12- to 24-h intervals to a maximum of 5 mg every 6 h.[16]

[b] Fenoldopam may increase intraocular pressure; administer with caution in patients with glaucoma or intraocular hypertension.

[c] Trimethaphan is a ganglionic blocker as well as a direct vasodilator.

TABLE 1.11

Therapeutic Considerations for End-Organ Complications of Hypertensive Emergencies[1,16-18]

Conditions	Preferred Treatments	Drugs to Avoid
Acute aortic dissection	Combination of a vasodilator and a beta-blocker (e.g., nitroprusside and esmolol)[a]; labetalol; trimethaphan[b]	Isolated use of pure vasodilators such as hydralazine or diazoxide
Cerebral infarction[c] or hemorrhage[d]	Use of antihypertensive therapy is controversial[c,d] Labetalol, nicardipine, or fenoldopam may be considered when treatment is indicated; nitroprusside, which increases intracerebral pressure and has a narrow therapeutic index, should be used with caution	Nitroglycerin or hydralazine (may increase intracranial pressure); diazoxide (may decrease cerebral blood flow); centrally acting agents (e.g., clonidine, methyldopa)
Hypertensive encephalopathy	Labetalol, nicardipine, or fenoldopam; nitroprusside, which increases intracerebral pressure and has a narrow therapeutic index, should be used with caution	Centrally acting agents (e.g., clonidine, methyldopa); diazoxide (may decrease cerebral blood flow)
Acute heart failure	Diuretics and ACE inhibitors (e.g., enalaprilat); nitroglycerin; nitroprusside	Nicardipine; beta-blockers (e.g., labetalol, esmolol)
Acute myocardial ischemia	Labetalol or esmolol in combination with nitroglycerin; nicardipine or fenoldopam may be added if pressure is not controlled with labetalol or esmolol alone	Isolated use of pure vasodilators such as hydralazine or diazoxide (may cause reflex tachycardia and increase myocardial oxygen demand); phentolamine; nicardipine; enalaprilat; nitroprusside (may decrease regional blood flow)
Acute renal failure	Fenoldopam; nicardipine	Diuretics or ACE inhibitors (use with caution); nitroprusside (thiocyanate and cyanide intoxication); nitroglycerin

TABLE 1.11 (CONTINUED)
Therapeutic Considerations for End-Organ Complications of Hypertensive Emergencies[1,16-18]

Conditions	Preferred Treatments	Drugs to Avoid
Eclampsia[e]	Hydralazine (traditional); labetalol or nicardipine is preferred in the intensive care unit	Nitroprusside; ACE inhibitors (contraindicated in pregnancy)
Sympathetic crisis[f]	Nicardipine, verapamil, or fenoldopam; phentolamine and nitroprusside are alternative agents	Beta-blockers (use of beta-blockers may lead to unopposed alpha-adrenergic vasoconstriction and a further rise in blood pressure)

[a] Because nitroprusside can cause reflex tachycardia, therapy with beta-blocker should be initiated beforehand. Metoprolol may be used as an alternative to esmolol. Nicardipine or fenoldopam is a less toxic alternative to nitroprusside.[16]

[b] Trimethaphan may be used when nitroprusside or beta-blocker is ineffective or poorly tolerated.

[c] Hypertension in the setting of acute ischemic stroke should be treated only "rarely and cautiously" according to the recommendations of the American Heart Association.[16] It is generally recommended that antihypertensive therapy be reserved for patients with a diastolic pressure >120 to 130 mm Hg, aiming to reduce the pressure by no more than an arbitrary figure of 20% in the first 24 h.[16]

[d] A recent study demonstrated that rapid reduction in blood pressure within the first 24 h after an intracerebral hemorrhage was associated with increased mortality. Therefore, careful and gradual lowering of a systolic blood pressure >200 mm Hg or a diastolic blood pressure >120 mm Hg is generally suggested when there is radiologic evidence of a major intracerebral bleed.[16]

[e] Parenteral magnesium is the treatment of choice to prevent the evolution of pre-eclampsia to eclampsia (seizures and worsening encephalopathy) in addition to delivery of the baby and placenta.[16,18]

[f] If sympathetic crisis is caused by abrupt discontinuation of sympathetic blockers such as clonidine or propranolol, control of blood pressure can usually be achieved by readministration of the discontinued drug.

ACE = angiotensin-converting enzyme.

REFERENCES

1. Joint National Committee on Prevention, Detection, Evaluation, and Treatment of High Blood Pressure. The Sixth Report of the Joint National Committee on Prevention, Detection, Evaluation, and Treatment of High Blood Pressure (JNC VI). *Arch Intern Med.* 1997;157:2413–2446.

2. Carretero OA, Oparil S. Essential hypertension: Part II: Treatment. *Circulation.* 2000;101:446–453.

3. Graves JW. Management of difficult to control hypertension. *Mayo Clin Proc.* 2000;75:278–284.

4. Smith SC Jr et al. AHA/ACC guidelines for preventing heart attack and death in patients with atherosclerotic cardiovascular disease: 2001 update. A statement of healthcare professionals from the American Heart Association and the American College of Cardiology. *J Am Coll Cardiol.* 2001;38:1581–1583.

5. Appel LJ et al. A clinical trial of the effects of dietary patterns on blood pressure: DASH Collaborative Research Group. *New Engl J Med.* 1997;336:1117–1124.

6. Frishman WH, Cheng-Lai A, Chen J, eds. *Current Cardiovascular Drugs,* 3rd ed. Philadelphia: Current Medicine; 2000.

7. Antihypertensive Therapy and Lipid Lowering Heart Attack Trial (ALLHAT) Collaborative Research Group. Major cardiovascular events in hypertensive patients randomized to doxazosin vs chlorthalidone: the Antihypertensive and Lipid-Lowering Treatment to Prevent Heart Attack Trial (ALLHAT). *J Am Med Assoc.* 2000;283:1967–1975.

8. Cheng A, Frishman WH. Use of angiotensin-converting enzyme inhibitors as monotherapy and in combination with diuretics and calcium channel blockers. *J Clin Pharmacol.* 1998;38:477–491.

9. Grossman E, Messerli FH, Neutel JM. Angiotensin II receptor blockers: equal or preferred substitutes for ACE inhibitors? *Arch Intern Med.* 2000;160:1905–1911.

10. World Health Organization–International Society of Hypertension guidelines for the management of hypertension. Guidelines Subcommittee. *J Hypertens.* 1999;17:151–183.

11. Lüscher TF, Cosentino F. The classification of calcium antagonists and their selection in the treatment of hypertension: a reappraisal. *Drugs.* 1998;55:509–517.

12. O'Rorke JE, Richardson WS. Evidence based management of hypertension: what to do when blood pressure is difficult to control. *Br Med J.* 2001;322:1229–1232.

13. Freis ED. Improving treatment effectiveness in hypertension. *Arch Intern Med.* 1999;159:2517–2521.

14. Jones D et al. Managing hypertension in the southeastern United States: applying the guidelines from the Sixth Report of the Joint National Committee on Prevention, Detection, Evaluation, and Treatment of High Blood Pressure (JNC VI). *Am J Med Sci.* 1999;318:357–364.

15. Moser M. Is it time for a new approach to the initial treatment of hypertension? *Arch Intern Med.* 2001;161:1140–1144.

16. Varon J, Marik PE. The diagnosis and management of hypertensive crises. *Chest.* 2000;118:214–227.
17. Bales A. Hypertensive crisis: how to tell if it's an emergency or an urgency. *Postgrad Med.* 1999;105:119–130.
18. Vaughan CJ, Delanty N. Hypertensive emergencies. *Lancet.* 2000;356:411–417.

2 Hyperlipidemia

Judy W.M. Cheng

CONTENTS

Step 1: Determine complete fasting lipid profile (9–12 h fast). If patients are not fasting, only total cholesterol and high-density lipoprotein (HDL).

Step 2: Identify presence of clinical atherosclerotic disease that confers high risk for coronary heart diseases (CHD) or CHD equivalent:
- Clinical CHD
- Symptomatic carotid artery disease
- Peripheral arterial disease
- Abdominal aortic aneurysm

Step 3: Determine presence of major risk factors (other then LDL):
- Cigarette smoking
- Hypertension (blood pressure > 140/90 mm Hg or receiving antihypertensive medications)
- Low HDL (<40 mg/dl)
- Family history of premature CHD (CHD in male first degree relative < 55 years and female first degree relative <65 years)
- Age (male >45 years, female >55 years)

Step 4: If 2+ risk factors (other than LDL) are present without CHD or CHD equivalent, assess 10-year (short-term) CHD risk (see Table 2.1, Framingham Point Scores).
The three levels of 10 year risk are as follows:
- >20% – CHD equivalent
- 10 to 20%
- <10%

Step 5: Establish LDL goal (see Table 2.2).

Step 6: Determine need for therapeutic lifestyle changes (TLC) (see Table 2.3).

Step 7: Determine need for drug consideration (see Table 2.2).

Step 8: Identify and treat metabolic syndrome and treat, if present, after 3 months of TLC (see Table 2.4).

Step 9: Treat elevated triglyceride and low HDL (see Figure 2.2).

FIGURE 2.1 Evaluation of patients with hyperlipidemia.

TABLE 2.1
Framingham Point Scores (estimate of 10-year risk)

Men		Women	
Age			
Age	Points	Age	Points
20–34	–9	20–34	–7
35–39	–4	35–39	–3
40–44	0	40–44	0
45–49	3	45–49	3
50–54	6	50–54	6
55–59	8	55–59	8
60–64	10	60–64	10
65–69	11	65–69	12
70–74	12	70–74	14
75–79	13	75–79	16

Total Cholesterol

Total Chol (mg/dl)	Points					Total Chol (mg/dl)	Points				
	Age (30–39)	Age (40–49)	Age (50–59)	Age (60–69)	Age (70–79)		Age (30–39)	Age (40–49)	Age (50–59)	Age (60–69)	Age (70–79)
<160	0	0	0	0	0	<160	0	0	0	0	0
160–199	4	3	2	1	0	160–199	4	3	2	1	1
200–239	7	5	3	1	0	200–239	8	6	4	2	1
240–279	9	6	4	2	1	240–279	11	8	5	3	2
≥280	11	8	5	3	1	≥280	13	10	7	4	2

Smoking

	Age (30–39)	Age (40–49)	Age (50–59)	Age (60–69)	Age (70–79)		Age (30–39)	Age (40–49)	Age (50–59)	Age (60–69)	Age (70–79)
Non-smoker	0	0	0	0	0	Non-smoker	0	0	0	0	0
Smoker	8	5	3	1	1	Smoker	9	7	4	2	1

TABLE 2.1 (CONTINUED)
Framingham Point Scores (estimate of 10-year risk)

Men		Women	

HDL

HDL (mg/dl)	Points	HDL (mg/dl)	Points
≥60	–1	≥60	–1
50–59	0	50–59	0
40–49	1	40–49	1
<40	2	<40	2

Systolic Blood Pressure (BP)

Systolic BP (mm Hg)	If Untreated	If Treated	Systolic BP (mm Hg)	If Untreated	If Treated
<120	0	0	<120	0	0
120–129	0	1	120–129	1	3
130–139	1	2	130–139	2	4
140–159	1	2	140–159	3	5
≥160	2	3	≥160	4	6

Point Total

Point Total	10-year Risk %	Point Total	10-year Risk %
<0	<1	<9	<1
0	1	9	1
1	1	10	1
2	1	11	1
3	1	12	1
4	1	13	2
5	2	14	2
6	2	15	3
7	3	16	4
8	4	17	5
9	5	18	6
10	6	19	8
11	8	20	11
12	10	21	14
13	12	22	17

TABLE 2.1 (CONTINUED)
Framingham Point Scores (estimate of 10-year risk)

Point Total (Continued)			
Point Total	10-year Risk %	Point Total	10-year Risk %
14	16	23	22
15	20	24	27
16	25	≥25	≥30
≥17	≥30		

TABLE 2.2
LDL Goals and Cutpoints for TLC and Drug Therapy in Different Risk Categories

Risk Category	LDL Goal (mg/dl)	LDL Level at Which to Initiate TLC (mg/dl)	LDL Level at Which to Consider Drug Therapy
CHD or CHD equivalents (10-year risk >20%)	<100	≥100	≥130 mg/dl (100–129 mg/dl, drug optional)
2+ risk factors (10-year risk ≤20%)	<130	≥130	10-year risk 10–20%: ≥130 mg/dl 10-year risk <10%: ≥160 mg/dl
0–1 risk factors[a]	<160	≥160	≥190 mg/dl (160–189 mg/dl: LDL-lowering drug optional)

[a] Patients with 0–1 risk factors will always turn out to have 10-year risk <10%; therefore assessment of risk score is not necessary.

TABLE 2.3
Initiation of TLC

TLC Feature:
• TLC diet (see below)
• Weight management
• Increase physical activities

Nutrient	Recommended Intake
Saturated fat	<7% of total calories
Polyunsaturated fat	Up to 10% of total calories
Monounsaturated fat	Up to 20% of total calories
Total fat	25–35% of total calories
Carbohydrate	50–60% of total calories
Fiber	20–30 g/day
Protein	Approximately 15% of total calories
Cholesterol	<200 mg/day
Total cholesterol	Balance energy intake and expenditure to maintain desirable body weight/weight weight gain

TABLE 2.4
Clinical Identification of the Metabolic Syndrome after 3 months of TLC

Metabolic Syndrome Is Defined as the Presence of Any THREE of the Following:

Risk Factors	Defining Level
Abdominal obesity	Waist circumference
Men	>102 cm (>40 in)
Women	>88 cm (>35 in)
Triglycerides	>150 mg/dl
HDL cholesterol	
Men	<40 mg/dl
Women	<50 mg/dl
Blood pressure	>130/85 mm Hg
Fasting glucose	>110 mg/dl

Treatment: aggressive weight control and physical activities.

TABLE 2.5
Antihyperlipidemic Therapy

Drug	LDL (%)	VLDL (%)	HDL (%)	Effects on Lipid	Monitoring Parameters	Comments
Bile Acid Sequestrants (BAS) Cholestyramine Cholestipol	↓15–30	↑5	↑3–5	↓LDL ↑LDL	Efficacy: Lipid panel 6–8 weeks after initiating therapy or every time doses are changed Once cholesterol profile achieved goal, repeat lipid profile every year Side effects: Constipation Space 4 h apart from other medication to prevent binding Monitor increase in triglyceride after 6–8 weeks of initiating therapy	Problem with compliance (need multiple daily doses)
Niacin	↓5–25	↓20–50	↑15–35	↓VLDL and LDL ↑HDL	Efficacy: Same as BAS Side effects: Flushing Liver toxicity Hyperglycemia Hyperuricemia, precipitate gout Exacerbate peptic ulcer disease	Problems with patient compliance due to intolerance; administer with ASA to minimize flushing

	↓5–20	↓20–50	↑10–20		
Fibric Acid	↓5–20	↓20–50	↑10–20	↓↓VLDL and LDL ↑HDL	Efficacy: Same as BAS Side effects: Liver toxicity Myopathy
Clofibrate					
Gemfibrozil					
Fenofibrate					
HMG-CoA reductase inhibitors (Statins)				↓↓LDL ↓HDL	Efficacy: Same as BAS Side effects: Liver toxicity Myopathy
Fluvastatin	↓24	↓10	↑8		
Pravastatin	↓34	↓24	↑12		
Lovastatin	↓34	↓16	↑9		
Simvastatin	↓41	↓18	↑12		
Atorvastatin	↓50	↓29	↑6		

ASA = aspirin

ATP III Classification of Serum Triglycerides (mg/dl)

<150	Normal
150 – 199	Borderline high
200 – 499	High
>500	Very high

Treatment of elevated triglycerides (150 mg/dl)

- Primary aim of therapy is to reach LDL goal.
- Intensify weight management.
- Increase physical activity.
- If triglycerides are 200 mg/dl after LDL goal is reached, set secondary goal for non-HDL cholesterol (total – HDL) 30 mg/dl higher than LDL goal.

Comparison of LDL Cholesterol and Non-HDL Cholesterol Goals for Three Risk Categories

Risk Category	LDL Goal (mg/dl)	Non-HDL Goal (mg/dl)
CHD and CHD Risk Equivalent (10-year risk for CHD >20%)	<100	<130
Multiple (2+) Risk Factors (10-year risk 20%)	<130	<160
0–1 Risk Factor	<160	<190

If triglycerides 200 – 499 mg/dl after LDL goal is reached, consider adding drug if needed to reach non-HDL goal:

- Intensify therapy with LDL-lowering drug, or
- Add nicotinic acid or fibrate to further lower VLDL.

If triglycerides 500 mg/dl, first lower triglycerides to prevent pancreatitis:

- Very low-fat diet (15% of calories from fat)
- Weight management and physical activity
- Fibrate or nicotinic acid
- When triglycerides <500 mg/dl, turn to LDL-lowering therapy

Treatment of low HDL cholesterol (<40 mg/dl)

- First reach LDL goal, then
- Intensify weight management and increase physical activity.
- If triglycerides 200 – 499 mg/dl, achieve non-HDL goal.
- If triglycerides <200 mg/dl (isolated low HDL) in CHD or CHD equivalent, consider nicotinic acid or fibrate.

FIGURE 2.2 Treating Elevated Triglycerides and Decreased HDL.

REFERENCES

1. Expert Panel on Detection, Evaluation, and Treatment of High Blood Cholesterol in Adults. Executive summary of the third report of the National Cholesterol Education Program (NCEP) expert panel on detection, evaluation and treatment of high blood cholesterol in adults (Adult Treatment Panel III). *J Am Med Assoc.* 2001;285(19):2486–2497.
2. Knopp RH. Drug therapy: drug treatment in lipid disorders. *New Engl J Med.* 1999;341:498–511.

3 Pharmacologic Management of Chronic Stable Angina

James Nawarskas

CONTENTS

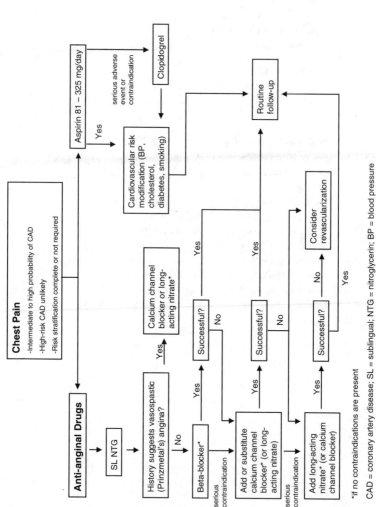

FIGURE 3.1 Pharmacologic management of chronic stable angina. (Adapted from Gibbons, R.J. et al., *Circulation*, 99, 2829, 1999.)

*If no contraindications are present

CAD = coronary artery disease; SL = sublingual; NTG = nitroglycerin; BP = blood pressure

TABLE 3.1
Select Pharmacologic and Pharmacokinetic Characteristics of Beta-Adrenergic Antagonists Used for the Treatment of Angina Pectoris[1-3]

Drug	FDA-Approved Indications	Adrenergic Receptor-Blocking Activity[a]	% Oral Bioavailability	Half-Life (h)	% Excreted Unchanged in Urine	Lipid Solubility[b]
Atenolol (Tenormin)	Hypertension, angina pectoris, acute MI	β_1	50–60	6–7	50 (PO), 85 (IV)	Low
Betaxolol (Kerlone)	Hypertension	β_1	89	14–22	15	Low
Bisoprolol (Zebeta)	Hypertension	β_1	80	9–12	50	Low
Labetalol (Trandate, Normodyne)	Hypertension	β_1,β_2,α_1	25–35	6–8	5	Moderate
Metoprolol (Lopressor, Toprol-XL)	Hypertension, angina pectoris, acute MI, heart failure (Toprol-XL only)	β_1	40–50 (IR), 77 (Toprol-XL)	3–7	<5 (PO), 10 (IV)	Moderate
Nadolol (Corgard)	Hypertension, angina pectoris	β_1,β_2	30–50	20–24	70	Low
Propranolol (Inderal, Inderal-LA)	Hypertension, angina pectoris, arrhythmias, post-MI prophylaxis	β_1,β_2	30 (IR), 9–18 (SR)	3–5 (IR), 8–11 (SR)	<1	High
Timolol (Blocadren)	Hypertension, post-MI prophylaxis	β_1,β_2	75	4	20	Low/moderate

[a] Indicates relative selectivity; all β-blockers act at both β_1 and β_2 receptors to some extent.
[b] It has been hypothesized that higher lipid solubility *may* result in greater central nervous system side effects.
FDA = U.S. Food and Drug Administration, PO = oral, IV = intravenous, IR = immediate-release, SR = sustained-release, MI = myocardial infarction.

TABLE 3.2
Dosing Characteristics of Beta-Adrenergic Antagonists Used in the Treatment of Angina Pectoris[1-3]

Drug	Availability	Usual Starting Dosage	Maximum Dosage (oral)
Atenolol (Tenormin)	25, 50, 100 mg tablets; 0.5 mg/ml injection	PO: 50 mg once daily IV: 5 mg × 2, 10 min apart	200 mg once daily
Betaxolol (Kerlone)	10, 20 mg tablets	5–10 mg once daily	40 mg once daily
Bisoprolol (Zebeta)	5, 10 mg tablets	2.5–5 mg once daily	20 mg once daily
Labetalol (Trandate, Normodyne)	100, 200, 300 mg tablets; 5 mg/ml injection	PO: 100 mg twice daily IV bolus: 20 mg, then 40–80 mg every 10 min as needed up to a total of 300 mg IV infusion: 2 mg/min up to a total of 300 mg	2400 mg/day in 2–3 divided doses
Metoprolol (Lopressor, Toprol-XL)	50, 100 mg tablets; 25, 50, 100, 200 mg SR tablets (Toprol XL); 1 mg/mL injection	PO IR: 50 mg twice daily; Toprol-XL: 50–100 mg once daily; 12.5–25 mg once daily for heart failure IV: 5 mg every 2 min. × 3 doses	450 mg/day; 400 mg/day Toprol-XL; 200 mg Toprol-XL for heart failure
Nadolol (Corgard)	20, 40, 80, 120, 160 mg tablets	40 mg once daily	240 mg once daily
Propranolol (Inderal)	10, 20, 40, 60, 80, 90 mg IR tablets; 60, 80, 120, 160 mg SR capsules (Inderal LA); 4 mg/ml, 8 mg/ml, 80 mg/ml oral solution; 1 mg/ml injection	PO IR: 40 mg twice daily PO SR: 80 mg once daily IV: 1 mg every 5 min to a maximum of 0.15 mg/kg	640 mg/day (hypertension); 320 mg/day (angina); 240 mg/day (MI)
Timolol (Blocadren)	5, 10, 20 mg tablets	10 mg twice daily	30 mg twice daily (hypertension) 10 mg twice daily (MI)

PO = oral, IV = intravenous, IR = immediate-release, SR = sustained release, MI = myocardial infarction.

TABLE 3.3
Select Pharmacologic and Pharmacokinetic Characteristics of Calcium Channel Antagonists[1-3]

Drug	Myocardial Contractility	Heart Rate	AV Nodal Conduction	Vascular Resistance	Oral Bioavailability, %	Half-Life (h)
Amlodipine (Norvasc)	↑/0	0	0	↓↓	64–90	30–50
Bepridil (Vascor)	0/↓	0/↓	0/↓	↓	59	26–64
Diltiazem (Cardizem, Dilacor XR, Tiazac)	↓	↓	↓	↓	38 (first-dose), 90 (long-term)	4–7
Felodipine (Plendil)	↑/0	↑/0	0	↓↓	20	11–16
Isradipine (DynaCirc)	↑/0	0/↑	0	↓↓	15–24	8
Nicardipine (Cardene)	↑/0	0/↑	0	↓↓	35	2–4
Nifedipine (Procardia XL, Adalat CC)	↓/0/↑	0/↑	0	↓↓	45–70	2–5
Nimodipine (Nimotop)	↑/0	0/↑	0	↓↓	13	1–2
Nisoldipine (Sular)	↑/0	0/↑	0	↓↓	5	7–12
Verapamil (Calan, Isoptin, Verelan)	↓↓	↓	↓↓	↓	20–35	3–7; may be up to 12 with multiple dosing

↓ = decrease, 0 = no change, ↑ = increase, ↓↓ = pronounced decrease.

AV = atrioventricular

TABLE 3.4

Dosing Characteristics of Calcium Channel Antagonists[1-3]

Drug	FDA-Approved Indications	Availability	Usual Starting Dosage[a]	Maximum Dosage[a]
Amlodipine (Norvasc)	Hypertension, chronic stable angina, vasospastic angina	2.5, 5, 10 mg tablets	5 mg once daily	10 mg once daily
Bepridil (Vascor)	Chronic stable angina unresponsive to other antianginal therapies	200, 300 mg tablets	200 mg once daily	400 mg once daily
Diltiazem (Cardizem, Dilacor XR, Tiazac; Cartia XT, Diltia XT	Hypertension, chronic stable angina, vasospastic angina, atrial tachyarrhythmias	30, 60, 90 120 mg IR tablet; 60, 90 120 mg SR (12-h) capsule (Cardizem SR); 120, 180, 240, 300, 360 mg SR (24-h) capsule; mg/ml injection	IR: 30–60 mg q6–8h Cardizem SR: 60–120 mg twice daily; 24-hour formulations: 120–180 mg once daily	480 mg/day
Felodipine (Plendil)	Hypertension	2.5, 5, 10 mg SR tablet	5 mg once daily	20 mg once daily
Isradipine (DynaCirc)	Hypertension	2.5, 5 mg IR capsules; 5, 10 mg SR capsules	IR: 2.5 mg BID SR: 5 mg once daily	IR: 10 mg BID SR: 20 mg once daily
Nicardipine (Cardene)	Chronic stable angina, (IR) hypertension (IR/SR)	20, 30 mg IR capsules; 30, 45, 60 mg SR capsules; 2.5 mg/ml injection	IR: 20 mg TID SR: 30 mg BID	IR: 40 mg TID SR: 60 mg BID

TABLE 3.4 (CONTINUED)
Dosing Characteristics of Calcium Channel Antagonists[1-3]

Drug	FDA-Approved Indications	Availability	Usual Starting Dosage[a]	Maximum Dosage[a]
Nifedipine (Procardia XL, Adalat CC, Nifedical XL)	Vasospastic angina, chronic stable angina, hypertension	10, 20 mg IR capsules[b] 30, 60, 90 mg SR tablet	30–60 mg once daily (SR)	120 mg once daily (SR)
Nimodipine (Nimotop)	Improvement of neurologic deficits secondary to subarachnoid hemorrhage (SAH)	30 mg capsule	Begun within 96 h of SAH: 60 mg q4h × 21 days	—
Nisoldipine (Sular)	Hypertension	10, 20, 30, 40 mg SR tablet	10–20 mg once daily	60 mg once daily
Verapamil (Calan, Isoptin SR, Verelan, Covera-HS)	Vasospastic angina, chronic stable angina, unstable angina, atrial tachyarrhythmias, hypertension	40, 80, 120 mg IR tablet; 120, 180, 240 mg SR tablet; 100, 120, 180, 200, 240, 300, 360 mg SR capsule; 2.5 mg/ml injection	IR: 40–120 mg TID SR: 120–240 mg once daily; Covera-HS and Verelan PM should be administered at bedtime	480 mg/day

[a] When multiple indications are present, antianginal dosage is provided.

[b] Use of IR nifedipine not recommended due to adverse events associated with its use.

SR = sustained-release, IR = immediate-release, BID = twice daily, TID = thrice daily.

TABLE 3.5

Monitoring Parameters, Adverse Effects, and Contraindications for Antianginal Drugs[1-3]

Drug/Drug Class	Monitoring Parameters	Common Adverse Effects	Contraindications
Beta-blockers	BP, HR (goal 50–60 bpm), angina symptoms, CNS adverse effects, signs/symptoms of heart failure, pulmonary compromise (bronchoconstriction), or peripheral vascular disease	Hypotension, bradycardia, lethargy/fatigue, poor exercise tolerance, loss of libido, depression, nightmares, insomnia (CNS side effects may be more prominent with more lipophilic drugs), exacerbation of preexisting pulmonary disease, heart failure, or peripheral vascular disease	Severe obstructive pulmonary disease, severe heart failure, second- or third-degree heart block, severe sinus node disease, asthma or active allergic rhinitis
Diltiazem, Verapamil	BP, HR, angina symptoms, signs/symptoms of heart failure	Hypotension, bradycardia, dizziness, headache, flushing, edema, skin reactions, exacerbation of preexisting heart failure, constipation, AV block	Second- or third-degree heart block, severe heart failure, severe sinus node disease, acute MI and pulmonary congestion (diltiazem), hypotension (SBP <90 mm Hg), atrial fibrillation with an accessory AV pathway (verapamil)
Amlodipine, Felodipine, Isradipine, Nicardipine, Nifedipine, Nimodipine, Nisoldipine	BP, HR, angina symptoms, signs of peripheral edema	Dizziness, hypotension, flushing, headache, peripheral edema, tachycardia	Symptomatic hypotension, advanced aortic stenosis (nicardipine)

TABLE 3.5 (CONTINUED)
Monitoring Parameters, Adverse Effects, and Contraindications for Antianginal Drugs[1-3]

Drug/Drug Class	Monitoring Parameters	Common Adverse Effects	Contraindications
Bepridil	BP, HR, angina symptoms, WBC count, QT interval, ECG for ventricular ectopy, serum potassium	Shortness of breath, dizziness, nervousness, tremor, palpitations, nausea, asthenia, diarrhea, headache, QT prolongation, agranulocytosis (rare)	History of ventricular arrhythmias, uncompensated cardiac insufficiency, congenital QT prolongation, use with other drugs that prolong the QT interval, sick sinus syndrome, 2° or 3° heart block, hypotension (SBP <90 mmHg)
Nitrates	BP, HR, anginal frequency, headache, dizziness	Dizziness, headache, flushing, weakness, nausea/vomiting, palpitations, tachycardia, postural hypotension, contact dermatitis with transdermal patches	Severe anemia, severe hypotension or uncompensated hypovolemia, increased intracranial pressure, use of sildenafil, closed angle glaucoma, constrictive pericarditis, cardiac tamponade

BP = blood pressue, HR = heart rate, WBC = white blood cell, ECG = electrocardiogram, CNS = central nervous system, AV = atrioventricular, MI = myocardial infarction, SBP = systolic blood pressure.

TABLE 3.6
Dosing Characteristics of Available Nitrate Products[2,3]

Nitrate	Dosage Form	Onset	Duration	Usual Dosage
Amyl nitrite	Inhalant	0.5 min	3–5 min	0.3 ml prn
Nitroglycerin	IV	1–2 min	3–5 min	IV initially 10 µg/min, increased by 10 µg/min every 3–5 min until one or more of the following end points is achieved: • Symptoms resolve • 10% decrease in MAP if normotensive, 30% decrease if hypertensive, keeping SBP ≥90 mm Hg • Increase in HR >10 bpm (not exceeding 110 bpm)
	SL tablet	1–3 min	30–60 min	0.15–0.6 mg (1 tablet or 1–2 sprays) × 3 prn 5 min apart; if no relief, seek immediate medical attention
	Translingual spray	2 min	30–60 min	
	Transmucosal tablet	1–2 min	3–5 h	1–3 mg q3–5 h while awake
	Oral, SR	20–45 min	3–8 h	2.5–2.6 mg 2–4 times daily initially; increase prn up to 26 mg 4 times daily
	Topical ointment	30–60 min	2–12 h	Initially, 0.5 in. (7.5 mg NTG) every 8 h, increased prn up to 5 in. (75 mg NTG) every 4 h; usual dosage is 1–2 in. every 8 h
	Transdermal	30–60 min	Up to 24 h	0.2–0.8 mg patch applied for 12 h each day

TABLE 3.6 (CONTINUED)
Dosing Characteristics of Available Nitrate Products[2,3]

Nitrate	Dosage Form	Onset	Duration	Usual Dosage
Isosorbide dinitrate (Isordil, Sorbitrate)	SL	2–5 min	1–3 h	2.5–5 mg initially, increased prn
	Oral	20–40 min	4–6 h	5–20 mg 3–4 times daily initially, increased prn up to 40 mg 4 times daily
	Oral, SR	Up to 4 h	6–8 h	40 mg 2–3 times daily initially, increased prn up to 80 mg 2–3 times daily
Isosorbide mononitrate	Oral, IR (Monoket, Ismo)	30–60 min	12–14 h	20 mg BID, spaced 7 h apart
	Oral, SR (Imdur, Isotrate ER)	Up to 4 h	12–24 h	30–60 mg once daily initially, increased as needed to a maximum of 240 mg once daily

IV = intravenous, SL = sublingual, IR = immediate-release, SR = sustained release, MAP = mean arterial pressure, NTG = nitroglycerin, SBP = systolic blood pressure, HR = heart rate, BID = twice daily.

Source: Adapted from *Drug Facts and Comparisons*. St. Louis, MO: Facts and Comparisons; 2002. With permission.

REFERENCES

1. Product prescribing information.
2. *Drug Facts and Comparisons*. St. Louis, MO: Facts and Comparisons, 2002.
3. Anderson PO, Knoben JE, Troutman WG, eds. 10th ed. *Handbook of Clinical Drug Data*. New York: McGraw-Hill; 2002.
4. Gibbons RJ et al. ACC/AHA/ACP-ASIM guidelines for the management of patients with chronic stable angina: executive summary and recommendations: a report of the American College of Cardiology/American Heart Association Task Force on Practice Guidelines (Committee on Management of Patients with Stable Angina). *Circulation*. 1999;99:2829–2848.

4 Pharmacologic Management of Acute Coronary Syndromes

James Nawarskas

CONTENTS

TABLE 4.1
American College of Cardiology/American Heart Association Classification System[1]

Class	Explanation
Class I	Conditions for which there is evidence and/or general agreement that a given procedure or treatment is beneficial, useful, and effective
Class II	Conditions for which there is conflicting evidence and/or a divergence of opinion about the usefulness/efficacy of a procedure or treatment
Class IIa	Weight of evidence/opinion is in favor of usefulness/efficacy
Class IIb	Usefulness/efficacy is less well established by evidence/opinion
Class III	Conditions for which there is evidence and/or general agreement that a procedure/treatment is not useful/effective and in some cases may be harmful

TABLE 4.2
ACC/AHA Guidelines for the Treatment of USA or NSTEMI[1,2]*

Drug	Class I	Class IIa	Class IIb	Class III
Nitroglycerin	SL, followed by IV administration ASAP upon presentation; all patients should be given SL NTG upon hospital discharge	—	—	Within 24 h of sildenafil use
Morphine sulfate	IV if symptoms not relieved by NTG or when acute pulmonary congestion and/or severe agitation is present	—	—	—
Beta-blocker	IV ASAP if chest pain present, followed by long-term PO administration	—	—	—
Calcium channel blockers	Verapamil diltiazem or amlodipine in place of beta-blocker in patients with a contraindication to a beta-blocker in the absence of severe LV dysfunction or other contraindications	Long-acting oral agents for recurrent ischemia in the absence of contraindications and when beta-blockers and nitrates are fully used	1. Extended-release verapamil or diltiazem in place of a beta-blocker; immediate-release dihydropyridines in the presence of a beta-blocker 2. In NSTEMI, diltiazem may be given to patients without LV dysfunction, pulmonary congestion, or CHF; it may be added to standard therapy after the first 24 h and continued for 1 year	Immediate-release dihydropyridies in the absence of a beta-blocker

TABLE 4.2 (CONTINUED)
ACC/AHA Guidelines for the Treatment of USA or NSTEMI[1,2] *

Drug	Class I	Class IIa	Class IIb	Class III
ACE inhibitor	Acutely, when hypertension persists despite treatment with NTG and a beta-blocker in patients with LV dysfunction or CHF and chronically in patients with diabetes, LV dysfunction/CHF, or hypertension	All post-ACS patients	—	—
Oral antiplatelet drugs	1. Aspirin, administered ASAP and continued indefinitely 2. Clopidogrel in patients unable to take aspirin 3. In hospitalized patients for whom an early noninterventional approach is planned, clopidogrel should be added to aspirin ASAP on admission and administered for 1–9 months	—	—	Dipyridamole

4. In patients for whom a PCI is planned, clopidogrel should be started and continued for 1–9 months in patients who are not at high risk for bleeding 5. In patients taking clopidogrel in whom CABG is planned, if possible the drug should be withheld for at least 5 days, and preferably for 7 days prior to surgery			
Heparin	IV UFH or SQ LMWH in all patients	Enoxaparin is preferable to UFH unless CABG is planned within 24 h	—	—
Glycoprotein IIb/IIIa receptor antagonist	In combination with aspirin and heparin for patients in whom catheterization and PCI are planned. The glycoprotein IIb/IIIa antagonist may also be administered just prior to PCI.	1. Eptifibatide or tirofiban should be administered, in addition to aspirin and heparin, to patients with continuing ischemia, an elevated troponin or with other high-risk features in whom an invasive management strategy is not planned	Eptifibatide or tirofiban, in addition to aspirin and heparin, to patients without continuing ischemia who have no other high-risk features and in whom PCI is not planned	Abciximab administration in patients in whom PCI is not planned

TABLE 4.2 (CONTINUED)
ACC/AHA Guidelines for the Treatment of USA or NSTEMI[1,2] *

Drug	Class I	Class IIa	Class IIb	Class III
		2. A platelet glycoprotein IIb/IIIa antagonist should be administered to patients already receiving heparin, aspirin, and clopidogrel in whom catheterization and PCI are planned. The glycoprotein IIb/IIIa antagonist may also be administered just prior to PCI.	—	—
Lipid-lowering medications	1. HMG CoA reductase inhibitors as an adjunct to dietary modification in all post-ACS patients with LDL >125 mg/dl and to all patients with LDL >100 mg/dl after dietary modification	1. Gemfibrozil or niacin in patients with a HDL <40 mg/dL and a triglyceride level >200 mg/dL		

| 2. A fibrate or niacin if HDL <40 mg/dL | 2. HMG-CoA reductase inhibitors and diet for LDL >100 mg/dL begun 24–96 h after admission and continued at hospital discharge |

USA, unstable angina; CNS, central nervous system; NSTEMI, non-ST elevation myocardial infarction; NTG, nitroglycerin; SL, sublingual; IV, intravenous; ASAP, as soon as possible; PO, oral; LV, left ventricular; ACE, angiotensin-converting enzyme; CHF, congestive heart failure; HDL, high-density lipoprotein, ACS, acute coronary syndromes; UFH, unfractionated heparin; SQ, subcutaneous; LMWH, low-molecular-weight heparin; PCI, percutaneous coronary intervention; CABG, coronary artery bypass grafting; LDL, low-density lipoprotein.

* Recommendations provided assume absence of contraindications unless otherwise stated.

TABLE 4.3
Dosage, Contraindications, and Monitoring of Medications Used in the Treatment of ACS[1-5]

Drug	Usual Inpatient Dosage	Usual Outpatient Dosage	Contraindications	Monitoring
Nitroglycerin	SL 0.4 mg × 3 prn, 5 min apart; IV initially 10 µg/min, increased by 10 µg/min every 3–5 min until symptoms resolve or blood pressure response is noted	SL 0.4 mg × 3 prn, 5 min apart	Severe hypotension or uncompensated hypovolemia, severe anemia, increased intracranial pressure, use of sildenafil, closed angle glaucoma, constrictive pericarditis, cardiac tamponade	BP, HR, angina frequency, dizziness, headache
Isosorbide dinitrate	Initially, 5–20 mg (IR) 3–4 times daily, titrated up to response	10–40 mg q6h (IR) 40–80 mg 08–12h (SR)		
Isosorbide mononitrate	Initially, 20 mg twice daily, separated 7 h apart (IR) or 30–60 mg once daily (SR)	120—240 mg/day		
Morphine sulfate	1–5 mg IV every 5–30 min prn for symptom relief	—	Hypotension, respiratory depression, circulatory depression, acute asthma	Pain control, signs of respiratory depression, BP, constipation

Beta-blockers	Metoprolol: 5 mg IV q 5 min. × 3, followed by 25–50 mg PO q6h × 48 h; followed by 100 mg PO BID or 200 mg PO extended-release QD Propranolol: 0.5–1.0 mg IV, followed in 1–2 hrs by 40–80 mg PO q6–8 h Atenolol: 5 mg IV over 5 min, followed 5 min later by another 5 mg IV dose, followed 1–2 h. later by 50–100 mg PO once daily	Dosage required to maintain resting HR of 50–60 bpm Maximum daily dosages: Metoprolol: 450 mg (IR); 400 mg (SR) Atenolol: 200 mg Propranolol: 320 mg	Severe obstructive pulmonary disease, severe heart failure, second- or third-degree heart block, severe sinus node disease, asthma or active allergic rhinitis	HR, BP, ECG, auscultation for rales and bronchospasm, angina symptoms, CNS adverse effects, signs/symptoms of heart failure pulmonary compromise or peripheral vascular disease
Calcium channel blockers	Initial dosages: Amlodipine: 5 mg once daily Diltiazem: IR: 30–60 mg q6–8h; SR: 120–180 mg once daily Verapamil: IR: 80–120 mg TID, SR: 120–240 mg once daily	Amlodipine: 5–10 mg once daily Diltiazem: 120–360 mg SR once daily Verapamil: 120–480 mg SR once daily	Second- or third- degree heart block, severe heart failure, severe sinus node disease, acute MI and pulmonary congestion (diltiazem), atrial fibrillation with an accessory AV pathway (verapamil), advanced aortic stenosis (nicardipine) symptomatic hypotension	BP, HR, angina symptoms, signs/symptoms of heart failure, peripheral edema

TABLE 4.3 (CONTINUED)
Dosage, Contraindications, and Monitoring of Medications Used in the Treatment of ACS[1-5]

Drug	Usual Inpatient Dosage	Usual Outpatient Dosage	Contraindications	Monitoring
Aspirin	160–325 mg initially, chewed for rapid effect, followed by 75–325 mg daily	75–325 mg once daily	Hypersensitivity, active bleeding, severe bleeding risk	Signs/symptoms of bleeding
Clopidogrel	75 mg once daily; may load with 300–600 mg if rapid onset is desired	75 mg once daily	Active bleeding, severe bleeding risk	Signs/symptoms of bleeding
Ticlopidine	250 mg twice daily, may load with 500 mg if rapid onset is desired	250 mg twice daily	Active bleeding, severe bleeding risk, presence of hentropenia or thrombocytopenia, history of thrombotic thrombocytogenic purpura	Signs/symptoms of bleeding CBC at baseline, then every 2 weeks after initiation of therapy for the first 3 months, then periodically thereafter

| Unfractionated heparin | USA/NSTEMI: 60–70 U/kg bolus (maximum 5000 U) IV followed by 12–15 U/kg/hr IV infusion (maximum 1000 U/hr) titrated to an aPTT 1.5–2.5 times control. With alteplase, reteplase, or tenecteplase for AMI: 60 U/kg bolus (max 4000 U) at initiation of thrombolytic, then an initial maintenance dose of about 12 U/kg/h (max 1000 U/h); maintenance infusions should be titrated to an aPTT 1.5–2.0 × control and given for 48 h; administration >48 h should be considered in patients at high risk for systemic or venous thromboembolism | — | Active bleeding, severe bleeding risk, history of heparin-induced thrombocytopenia, severe thrombocytogenia | aPTT, daily hemoglobin/hematocrit and platelet counts; signs/symptoms of bleeding |

TABLE 4.3 (CONTINUED)
Dosage, Contraindications, and Monitoring of Medications Used in the Treatment of ACS[1-5]

Drug	Usual Inpatient Dosage	Usual Outpatient Dosage	Contraindications	Monitoring
	With streptokinase, anistreplase, or urokinase for AMI: Heparin should be withheld for 6 h, then an aPTT obtained; heparin should be started when the aPTT is <2.0 × control, then infused to keep the aPTT 1.5–2.0 × control (initial infusion rate about 1000 U/h); after 48 h, a change to SQ heparin, Warfarin, or aspirin alone should be considered			
Low-molecular-weight heparin	Enoxaparin: 1 mg/kg SQ q12h Dalteparin: 120 IU/kg (max. 10,000 IU) SQ q12h	—	Active major bleeding, history of heparin-induced thrombocytopenia	Signs/symptoms of bleeding; periodic platelet counts

| Glycoprotein IIb/IIIa receptor antagonists | Eptifibatide: 180 μg/kg IV bolus followed by 2 μg/kg/min × 72–96 h
Tirofiban: 0.4 μg/kg/min × 30 min IV followed by 0.1 μg/kg/min × 48–96 h | — | Active bleeding, severe bleeding risk, prior stroke, severe hypertension (SBP >200 mm Hg or DBP >110 mm Hg) not adequately controlled on antihypertensive therapy, major surgery within the preceding 6 weeks | Daily hemoglobin and platelet counts; signs/symptoms of bleeding |

ACS = acute coronary syndromes; SL = sublingual; BP = blood pressure; HR = heart rate; IR = immediate-release; SR = sustained-release; IV = intravenous; PO = oral; BID = twice daily; ECG = electrocardiogram; CNS = central nervous sysem; MI = myocardial infarction, AV = atrioventricular; TID = thrice daily; CBC = complete blood count; USA = unstable angina; NSTEMI = non-ST-elevation myocardial infarction; AMI = acute myocardial infarction; aPTT = activated partial thromboplastin time; SQ = subcutaneous; SBP = systolic blood pressure; DBP = diastolic blood pressure

TABLE 4.4
Initial Management of Acute Myocardial Infarction (AMI)[1,2] *

Drug	Class I	Class IIa	Class IIb	Class III
IV nitroglycerin	1. For the first 24–48 h in patients with AMI and CHF, large anterior infarction, persistent ischemia, or hypertension 2. Continued use (beyond 48 h) in patients with recurrent angina or persistent pulmonary congestion	—	1. For the first 24–48 h in all patients with AMI who do not have hypotension, bradycardia, or tachycardia 2. Continued use (beyond 48 h may substitute oral or topical preparations) in patients with a large or complicated infarction	1. SBP <90 mm Hg or HR <50 bpm 2. Within 24° of sildenafil use.
Oral antiplatelet agents	1. 160–325 mg of aspirin should be given on day 1 of AMI and continued indefinitely on a daily basis 2. Clopidogrel in patients unable to take aspirin	—		Dipyridamole

Thrombolytics	1. ST elevation >0.1 mV in ≥2 contiguous leads, time to therapy ≤12 h, age <75 yr 2. BBB (obscuring ST-segment analysis) and history suggesting MI	1. ST elevation, age ≥75 yr	1. ST elevation, time to therapy >12–24 h 2. SBP >180 mm Hg or DBP >110 mm Hg associated with high-risk MI	1. ST elevation, time to therapy >24 h; ischemic pain resolved 2. ST depression only 3. Absence of acute ST elevation, a true posterior MI, or a presumed new LBBB
Glycoprotein IIb/IIIa antagonists	STEMI = none NSTEMI = see Table 4.2	STEMI = none NSTEMI = see Table 4.2	STEMI = none NSTEMI = see Table 4.2	—
Heparin	1. Patients undergoing percutaneous or surgical revascularization	1. IV UFH in patients receiving t-PA	Patients treated with non-selective thrombolytics, not at high risk, SQ heparin 7500–12,500 units twice daily until completely ambulatory	Routine IV UFH within 6 h to patients receiving streptokinase, urokinase, or anistreplase who are not at high risk for systemic embolism

TABLE 4.4 (CONTINUED)
Initial Management of Acute Myocardial Infarction (AMI)[1,2] *

Drug	Class I	Class IIa	Class IIb	Class III
	2. IV UFH or SQ LMWH in patients with NSTEMI	2. SQ UFH or LMWH in all patients not treated with thrombolytic therapy and who do not have a contra-indication to heparin. In patients at high risk for systemic emboli (large or anterior MI, atrial fibrillation, previous embolus, or known LV thrombus), IV UFH is preferred 3. IV in patients treated with nonselective thrombolytics (strep-tokinse, anistreplase, urokinase) who are at high risk for systemic emboli		

Beta-blockers	1. All patients without a contraindication who can be treated within 12 h of onset of infarction	Patients with moderate LV failure (bibasilar rales without evidence of low cardiac output) or other relative contraindications to beta-blocker therapy, provided patients can be closely monitored	Severe LV failure
	2. Patients with continuing or recurrent ischemic pain		
	3. Patients with tachyarrhythmias, such as atrial fibrillation with a rapid ventricular response		
	4. NSTEMI		

4. Enoxagarin preferred to UFH for NSTEMI unless CABG is planned within 24°

—

TABLE 4.4 (CONTINUED)
Initial Management of Acute Myocardial Infarction (AMI)[1,2]*

Drug	Class I	Class IIa	Class IIb	Class III
ACE inhibitors	1. Patients within the first 24 h of AMI with ST elevation in ≥2 precordial leads or with clinical heart failure in the absence of hypotension (SBP <100 mm Hg) or known contraindications to ACE inhibitors 2. LVEF <40% or patients with clinical heart failure on the basis of systolic pump dysfunction during and after convalescence from AMI	1. All other patients within the first 24 h of suspected or established AMI		—

Calcium channel blockers	STEMI = none NSTEMI = see Table 4.2	STEMI = Verapamil or diltiazem may be given to patients in whom beta-blockers are ineffective or contraindicated for relief of ongoing ischemia or control of a rapid ventricular response with atrial fibrillation after AMI in the absence of CHF, LV dysfunction, or AV block NSTEMI = see Table 4.2	STEMI = none NSTEMI = see Table 4.2	1. Short-acting nifedipine 2. Diltiazem and verapamil in patients with AMI and associated LV dysfunction or CHF 3. All immediate-release dihydropyridines in the absence of a beta-blocker
Magnesium	—	STEMI = 1. Correction of magnesium (and/or potassium) deficits, especially in patients receiving diuretics before onset of infarction NSTEMI = see Table 4.2	Magnesium bolus and infusion in high-risk patients such as elderly individuals and/or those for whom reperfusion therapy is not suitable	—

TABLE 4.4 (CONTINUED)
Initial Management of Acute Myocardial Infarction (AMI)[1,2] *

Drug	Class I	Class IIa	Class IIb	Class III
		2. Episodes of torsade de pointes associated with a prolonged QT interval should be treated with 1–2 g of magnesium administered as a bolus over 5 min		

CHF = congestive heart failure, SBP = systolic blood pressure, HR = heart rate, BBB = Bundle branch block, LBBB = left bundle branch block, DBP = diastolic blood pressure, MI = myocardial infarction, STEMI = ST-elevation myocardial infarction, NSTEMI = non-ST-elevation myocardial infarction, UFH = unfractionated heparin, SQ = subcutaneous, LMWH = low-molecular-weight heparin, LV = left ventricular, CABG = coronary artery bypass grafting, ACE = angiotensin-converting enzyme, LVEF = left ventricular ejection fraction

* Recommendations provided assume absence of contraindications unless otherwise stated.

TABLE 4.5
Chronic Management of Myocardial Infarction[1,2,12]

Drug	Class I	Class IIa	Class IIb	Class III
Antiplatelet therapy	1. 160–325 mg of aspirin should be given on day 1 of AMI and continued indefinitely on a daily basis 2. Clopidogrel (preferred) or ticlopidine in patients unable to take aspirin	—		Dipyridamole
Lipid-lowering therapy	See Table 4.2	See Table 4.2	Niacin or gemfibrozil may be added to diet if triglycerides >200 mg/dl	—
Beta-blockers	All but low-risk patients without a contraindication; treatment should begin ASAP and continue indefinitely	Low-risk patients without a clear contraindication	Patients with moderate or severe LV failure or other relative contraindication, provided patients can be closely monitored	—

TABLE 4.5 (CONTINUED)
Chronic Management of Myocardial Infarction[1,2,12]

Drug	Class I	Class IIa	Class IIb	Class III
ACE inhibitors	Treat all patients indefinitely post MI; start early in stable high-risk patients (anterior MI, previous MI, Killip class II (S3gallop, rales, radiographic CHF); consider chronic therapy for all other patients with coronary or other vascular disease unless contraindicated	—	—	—
Warfarin	1. Secondary prevention of MI in post-MI patients unable to take aspirin 2. Post-MI patients with persistent atrial fibrillation 3. Patients with LV thrombus	1. Patients with extensive wall motion abnormalities 2. Patients with paroxysmal atrial fibrillation	Patients with severe LV systolic dysfunction with or without CHF	—

| Hormone replacement therapy (estrogen/ progestin) | — | 1. Should *not* be given *de novo* to postmenopausal women after AMI for secondary prevention of coronary events

2. Postmenopausal women who are already taking HRT at the time of MI may continue to take this therapy | — |

AMI = acute myocardial infarction, MI = myocardial infarction, ASAP = as soon as possible, LV = left ventricular, CHF = congestive heart failure, HRT = hormone replacement therapy

TABLE 4.6
Comparison of Unfractionated Heparin, Low-Molecular-Weight Heparin, and Bivalirudin[3,6]

	Unfractionated Heparin	Low-Molecular Weight Heparin	Bivalirudin
Predictability of anticoagulation	Poor	Good	Good
Laboratory monitoring	aPTT, platelet counts	Platelet counts	None
Administration	IV bolus + infusion or SQ bolus	SQ bolus	IV bolus + infusion
Half-life	Dose-dependent; average 60–90 min	3–5 h	25 min
Thrombocytopenia	5–10%	≤2%	Not reported
Effects on thrombin inhibition	Indirect effect; unable to neutralize clot-bound thrombin	Indirect effect; unable to neutralize clot-bound thrombin	Direct effect; inhibits both free and clot-bound thrombin
Clinical indications	Prevention and treatment of venous thromboembolism, treatment of unstable angina and acute MI; prevention of thromboembolic complications of percutaneous coronary intervention	Prevention and treatment of venous thromboembolism, treatment of unstable angina and acute MI	Prevention of thromboembolic complications of percutaneous coronary intervention

aPTT = activated partial thromboplastin time, IV = intravenous, SQ = subcutaneous, MI = myocardial infarction

TABLE 4.7
Comparison of Thrombolytic Drugs[3,5,8,10,11,13]

	SK 1.5 MU Over 1 h	APSAC 30 mg over 2–5 min	Alteplase (rt-PA) 15 mg bolus, then 0.75 mg/kg (max. 50 mg) over 30 min, then 0.5 mg/kg (max. 35 mg) over 60 min	Reteplase 10 + 10 U in 30 min	TNKase max. 50 mg over 5 s
Half-life (min)	18–23	70–120	3–8	15–18	18–20
Antigenic	Yes	Yes	No	No	No
Intracranial hemorrhage (%)	0.3	0.6	0.1–0.75	0.8	0.9
Patency at 90 min (%)	59	65	81	85	88
TIMI grade 3 flow at 90 min (%)	32	43	54	60	66
Preferred if duration of symptoms ≤6 h		✔			✔
Preferred if duration of symptoms ≤12 h	✔	✔	✔	✔	
Concomitant heparin usage			✔	✔	✔
Fibrin specificity	—	—	+ +	+	+ + +
Cost/dose ($)	300	1800	2200	2200	2200

SK = streptokinase, APSAC = anisoylated plasminogen-streptokinase activator complex, TNKase = tenecteplase

TABLE 4.8
Absolute and Relative Contraindications to Thrombolytic Therapy for Acute Myocardial Infarction[13]

Absolute

    Previous hemorrhagic stroke at any time; other strokes or cerebrovascular event within 1 y

    Known intracranial neoplasm

    Active internal bleeding (not including menses)

    Suspected aortic dissection

Relative

    Severe, uncontrolled hypertension on presentation (BP >180/110 mm Hg)

    History of prior cerebrovascular accident or known intracerebral pathology not covered in absolute contraindications

    Current use of anticoagulants in therapeutic doses (INR ≥3)

    Known bleeding diathesis

    Recent trauma (within 2–4 weeks), including head trauma or traumatic or prolonged (>10 min) CPR or major surgery (<3 weeks)

    Noncompressible vascular puncture

    Recent (within 2–4 weeks) internal bleeding

    For streptokinase or anistreplase, prior exposure (5 days to 2 years) or prior allergic reactions

    Pregnancy

    Active peptic ulcer

    History of severe, chronic hypertension

BP = blood pressure, INR = international normalized ratio, CPR = cardiopulmonary resuscitation

TABLE 4.9
Comparison of Glycoprotein IIb/IIIa Receptor Antagonists[3,7,8]

	Abciximab (ReoPro®)	Tirofiban (Aggrastat®)	Eptifibatide (Integrilin®)
Antigenic	Yes	No	No
Thrombocytopenia (platelet count <100,000)	2–6%	1.5%	1.2%
Duration of effect	Long	Short	Short
Renal elimination	No	Yes	Yes
Reversibility with platelets	Yes, with platelet transfusion; may take up to 12 h	No	No
Binds to vitronectin receptor[a]	Yes	No	No
Cost[b]	$1620–2160	$840–1700	$1800–2300

[a] The vitronectin receptor mediates the ability of platelets to coagulate and may control some of the proliferative properties of vascular endothelial and smooth muscle cells. This is currently of unknown clinical consequence.

[b] Average wholesale price for treatment of acute coronary syndromes (tirofiban, eptifibatide) or percutaneous intervention (abciximab) in 80 kg patient.

TABLE 4.10
Antithrombotic Therapy in Patients Undergoing Percutaneous Coronary Intervention[8,9]

Drug	Indication	Dosage
Aspirin	Pretreatment in most patients	80–325 mg daily
Clopidogrel/ Ticlopidine	1. Pretreatment in patients intolerant of aspirin 2. Adjunct to aspirin in patients undergoing coronary stent placement	Clopidogrel: 300 mg load, then 75 mg/day for 14–30 days Ticlopidine: 500 mg load, then 250 mg BID for ≥10–14 days after the procedure
GPIIb/IIIa receptor antagonists	All patients, especially those with refractory unstable angina or other high-risk features; abciximab is preferred for patients undergoing primary PCI for AMI	Abciximab: 0.25 mg/kg IV bolus followed by 0.125 μg/kg/min (max. 10 μg/min) for 12 h Eptifibatide: 180 μg/kg IV bolus followed by 2 μg/kg/min infusion followed by a second 180 μg/kg IV bolus 10 min. after the first with the infusion continued for 18–24 h
		Tirofiban: 0.4 μg/kg/min for 30 min. followed by 0.1 μg/kg/min infusion for 12–24 hr after the pocedure or 10 μg/kg bolus followed by 0.15 μg/kg/min infusion for 36 h
Heparin	All patients	IV to maintain an ACT of 250–300 s (HemoTec device) or 300–350 s (Hemochron device); when abciximab is administered, goal ACT of >200 s (either device) is recommended

TABLE 4.10 (CONTINUED)
Antithrombotic Therapy in Patients Undergoing Percutaneous Coronary Intervention[8,9]

Drug	Indication	Dosage
Bivalirudin	1. All patients as an alternative to heparin 2. Patients with a history of heparin-induced thrombocytopenia	IV bolus 1.0 mg/kg, followed by 2.5 mg/kg/h × 4 h. If desired, this may be followed by a 0.2 mg/kg/h infusion for up to 20 h

GP = glycoprotein, PCI = precutaneous coronary intervention, AMI = acute myocardial infarction, ACT = activated clotting time, IV = intravenous

REFERENCES

1. Ryan TJ et al. 1999 update: ACC/AHA Guidelines for the management of patients with acute myocardial infarction: executive summary and recommendations: a report of the American College of Cardiology/American Heart Association Task Force on Practice Guidelines (Committee on Management of Acute Myocardial Infarction). *Circulation* 1999;100:1016–1030.

2. Braunwald E et al. ACC/AHA guideline update for the management of patients with unstable angina and non-ST-segment elevation myocardial infarction: a report of the American College of Cardiology/American Heart Association Task Force on Practice Guidelines (Committee on the Management of Patients with Unstable Angina). 2002. Available at: *http://www.acc.org/clinical/guidelines/unstable/unstable.pdf*.

3. Product prescribing information.

4. Cairns JA et al. Antithrombotic agents in coronary artery disease. *Chest.* 2001;119(suppl):228S–252S.

5. Ohman EM et al. Intravenous thrombolysis in acute myocardial infarction. *Chest.* 2001;199(suppl):253S–277S.

6. Hirsh J et al. Heparin and low-molecular-weight heparin: mechanisms of action, pharmacokinetics, dosing, monitoring, efficacy, and safety. *Chest.* 2001;119(suppl):64S–94S.

7. *Drug Topics Red Book* 2002. Montvale, NJ, Medical Economics Company, Inc.; 2002.

8. Spinler SA. Acute coronary syndromes. In: *Pharmacotherapy Self-Assessment Program* (PSAP), Book 1. 4th ed. American College of Clinical Pharmacy, St. Louis, MO. 2001.

9.   Popma JJ et al. Antithrombotic therapy in patients undergoing percutaneous coronary intervention. *Chest.* 2001;199(suppl):321S–336S.

10. Anderson PO, Knoben JE, Troutman WG, eds. *Handbook of Clinical Drug Data.* 10th ed. New York: McGraw-Hill, 2002.

11. Meister FL et al. Thrombolytic therapy for acute myocardial infarction. *Pharmacotherapy.* 1998;18:686–698.

12. Smith SC Jr et al. AHA/ACC Guidelines for Preventing Heart Attack and Death in Patients with Atherosclerotic Cardiovascular Disease: 2001 Update. *Circulation* 2001;104:1577–1579.

13. Ryan TJ et al. ACC/AHA guidelines for the management of patients with acute myocardial infarction: 1999 update: a report of the American College of Cardiology/American Heart Association Task Force on Practice Guidelines. Available at *www.acc.org.* Accessed on June 8, 2002.

5 Acute and Chronic Systolic Heart Failure

Judy W.M. Cheng

CONTENTS

0-58716-044-7/03/$0.00+$1.50

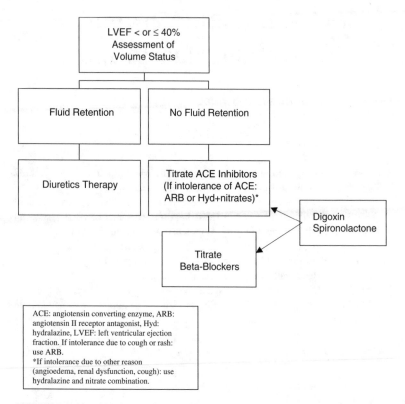

FIGURE 5.1 Algorithm in chronic heart failure management.[1] ACE: angiotensin converting enzyme, ARB: angiotensin II receptor antagonist, Hyd: hydralazine, LVEF: left ventricular ejection fraction. *If intolerance due to cough or rash, use ARB. If intolerance due to other reason (angioedema, renal dysfunction, cough); use hydralazine and nitrate combination.

TABLE 5.1
Stepwise Approach in Diuresing Patients with Decompensated Heart Failure

Step 1	Eliminate any cause that may cause fluid retention. Then, initiate intravenous furosemide 20–80 mg IV × 1 based on patient's fluid status and blood pressure.
	Monitor urine output for the next 6 h (goal urine output: >60 ml/h)
Step 2	If response is desirable, repeat furosemide dose every 6–12 h if necessary, targeting for daily decrease in weight of 0.5–1 kg daily (may be more aggressive based on patient's fluid status).
Step 3	If response is undesirable, increase dose of furosemide every 6 h up to a single dose of 200 mg intravenously.
Step 4	If response continues to be undesirable, add metolazone 2.5 mg po to 10 mg po bid or Chlorothiazide IV 500 mg to 1 g qd to bid for synergistic effects.
	May also consider switching to a different loop diuretics (bumetinide).
Step 5	If response continues to be undesirable, may try continuous furosemide infusion (5–20 mg/h).
Step 6	Dialysis

Note: May need to consider adding acetazolamide therapy 250 mg po qd to qid if patients develop metabolic alkalosis with aggressive loop diuretics therapy (caution of serious hypokalemia). Nesiritide therapy may also be considered from steps 3 to 5.

TABLE 5.2

Medications Used in Heart Failure (see other tables specifically for ACE inhibitors and Digoxin)[5,6]

Drug	Initial Dose	Maximum Dose	Major Side Effects
Thiazide	25 mg po qd	50 mg po qd	Postural hypotension,
Hydrochlorothiazide	25 mg po qd	50 mg po qd	hypokalemia,
Chlorthalidone	500 mg IV qd	1 g IV bid	hypomagnesemia,
Chlorothiazide	2.5 mg po qd	10 mg po bid	hyponatremia,
Metolazone			hyperuricemia,
			hyperglycemia
Loop Diuretics[a]			
Furosemide	10 mg po/IV qd	240 mg po/IV bid	
Torsemide	10 mg po/IV qd	200 mg po/IV qd	
Bumetidnide	0.5 mg po/IV qd	10 mg po/IV qd	
Ethacrynic acid	50 mg po/IV qd	200 mg po bid (100 mg IV bid)	
Potassium Sparing Diuretics[b]			
Spironolactone	12.5 mg po qd	50 mg po qd	Hyperkalemia, gynecomastia
Angiotensin II Receptor Antagonists			Hyperkalemia, elevation of serum creatinine, angioedema
Losartan	25 mg po qd	100 mg po qd	
Candesartan	2 mg po qd	32 mg po qd	
Valsartan	80 mg qd	320 mg qd	
Irbesartan	150 mg qd	300 mg qd	
Hydralazine	10 mg po/IV tid	100 mg po/IV tid (target dose: 75 mg po/IV tid[6])	Headache, lupus (with long-term use only)
Nitrates			Headache, hypotension
Isosorbide dinitrate	10 mg po tid	80 mg po tid (target dose: 40 mg po tid[6])	
Isosorbide mononitrate			
Imdur	30 mg po qd	240 mg po qd	
ISMO	20 mg po bid	120 mg po bid	
IV nitroglycerin	5 µg/min	Titrate to effect	

TABLE 5.2 (CONTINUED)
Medications Used in Heart Failure (see other tables specifically for ACE inhibitors and Digoxin)[5,6]

Drug	Initial Dose	Maximum Dose	Major Side Effects
Natriuretic Peptide			
Nesiritide	2 μg/kg bolus, then 0.01 μg/kg/min	0.03 μg/kg/min	
Positive Inotropes			Tachycardia
Dobutamine	2.5 μg/kg/min	20 μg/kg/min	
Milrinone	0.375 μg/kg/min	0.75 μg/kg/min	
Vasopressors			Tachycardia
Dopamine			
Dopaminergic dose	1 μg/kg/min	3 μg/kg/min	
Beta-1 dose	4 μg/kg/min	10 μg/kg/min	
Alpha-1 dose	11 μg/kg/min	Titrate to effect	
Epinephrine	1 μg/min	4 μg//min	
Norepinephrine	8 μg/min	12 μg/min	
Phenylnephrine	0.1 mg/min	0.2 mg/min	
Vasopressin	0.02 units/min	0.1 units/min	

[a] For chronic heart failure management only. See Table 5.1 for acute heart failure management.

[b] Only spironolactone has been demonstrated beneficial for heart failure management. Dosage used in heart failure management is considerably lower than other indications of spironolactone.[7]

TABLE 5.3
Initiating and Dosing Angiotensin Converting Enzyme (ACE) Inhibitors[8-11]

Step 1	Initiate therapy with short-acting ACE inhibitor (i.e., Captopril).
	Incremental increase of doses if patient is not hypotensive after each dose: 6.25 mg po, then 12.5 mg in 8 h, then 25 mg po qd in 8 h, then 50 mg po q8h thereafter.
	If patient is hypotensive in any dosage initiated above, then take the dose back one step, and continue with that dose q8h.
Step 2	Once stabilized, switch patient over to long-acting, once daily ACE inhibitor to enhance compliance.
Step 3	If necessary for blood pressure control (goal of BP <130/85 mm Hg), increase ACE inhibitor up to maximum dose.

ACE Inhibitor	Starting Dose	Target Dose	Maximum Dose
Benazepril	5 mg po qd	NA	40 mg daily (one or two doses)
Captopril	6.25 mg po tid	50 mg po tid	100 mg po tid
Enalapril	2.5 mg po bid	10 mg po bid	20 mg po bid
Fosinopril	5 mg po qd	40 mg po qd	80 mg po qd
Lisinopril	5 mg po qd	20 mg po qd	40 mg po qd
Quinapril	5 mg po qd	20 mg po qd	40 mg po qd
Ramipril	2.5 mg po qd	5 mg po bid 10 mg po qd	20 mg po daily (one or two doses)

Step 4	For patients who cannot tolerate ACE inhibitors due to cough or rash, substitute with angiotensin II receptor antagonists (see doses in Table 5.1).
	For patients who cannot tolerate ACE inhibitors due renal dysfunction and hyperkalemia, substitute vasodilator therapy with hydralazine + nitrates (see doses in Table 5.1).

TABLE 5.4
Dosing and Managing Beta-Blocker Therapy in Heart Failure[12,13]

Step 1	Make sure patient is not having clinical heart failure symptoms. Start Carvedilol 3.125 mg po bid or metoprolol (sustained release) 25 mg po qd.
Step 2	For outpatient, double doses no more often than 2 weeks. For inpatients, can double dose more frequently under close supervision (provided patient tolerated).
Step 3	Target dose: Carvedilol: > 80 kg, 50 mg po bid; < 80 kg, 25 mg po bid Metoprolol sustained released (Toprol XL): 200 mg po qd

Note: Diuretic doses may need to be temporarily increased during the beta-blocker dose titration phase. Spacing the administration of ACE inhibitor and beta-blockers apart can prevent excessive hypotension.

TABLE 5.5
Digoxin Dose[1]

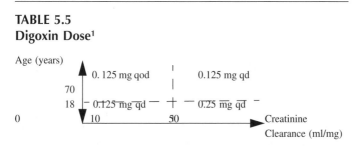

Dose applies to both IV and po. Dose is to be reduced a further 50% if patient is also on amiodarone, verapamil, quinidine.

TABLE 5.6
Patient Follow-Up by Pharmacists

Medications Issues to Be Discussed with Patients:
    Effects of medications on quality of life and survival
    Dosing of drugs
    Daily weight
    Likely side effects and what to do if they occur
    Coping mechanisms for complicated medical regimens
    Importance of compliance with treatment care plan
Dietary Recommendations:
    Sodium restriction
    Avoidance of excessive fluid intake
    Alcohol restriction, if appropriate
    Low fat diet
Avoid Medications That May Exacerbate Heart Failure:
    Antiarrhythmics (except amiodarone and dofetilide)
    Nonsteroidal anti-inflammatory agents
    Steroids
    Calcium channel blockers (except amlodipine and felodipine)[15,16]
    Anthracyclines
    Thiazolidinedione
Other Pharmacological Issues (to avoid):
    Inadequate ACE inhibitor therapy
    Suboptimal doses of vasodilators
    Ineffective diuretic regimen
    Excessive diuretics
    Discontinuation of digoxin in stable heart failure patients
    Not treating concurrent arrhythmias (both atrial and ventricular) appropriately
    Not preventing or treating hypokalemia, hypomagnesemia, and hyponatremia

REFERENCES

1. ACC/AHA Guidelines for Evaluation and Management of Chronic Heart Failure in the Adults. Available at: *http://www.americanheart.org/downloadable/heart/5360_HFGuidelineFinal.pdf.* Accessed 25 Jan 2002.
2. Haas GJ, Young JB. Acute heart failure management. In: Topol E, ed. *Textbook of Cardiovascular Medicine.* Philadelphia: Lippincott-Raven Publishers; 1998:2247–2271.

3. Rozenfeld V, Cheng JW. The role of vasopressin in the treatment of vasodilation in shock states. *Ann Pharmacother.* 2000;34(2):250–254.

4. Yelton SL, Gaylor MA, Murray KM. The role of continuous infusion loop diuretics. *Ann Pharmacother.* 1995;29(10):1010–1014.

5. Kastrup EK, ed. *Drug Facts and Comparison 2000.* 54th ed. St. Louis, MO: Wolters Kluwer Company; 2000.

6. Cohn JN et al. A comparison of enalapril with hydralazine-isosorbide in treatment of chronic congestive heart failure. *New Engl J Med.* 1991;325:303–310.

7. Pitt B et al. The effect of spironolactone on morbidity and mortality in patients with severe heart failure. Randomized aldactone evaluation study investigators. *New Engl J Med.* 1999;341(10):709–717.

8. Pfeffer MA et al. Effect of captopril on mortality and morbidity in patients with left ventricular dysfunction after myocardial infarction. Results of the survival and ventricular enlargement trial. The SAVE Investigators. *New Engl J Med.* 1992;327(10):669–677.

9. The SOLVD investigators. Effect of enalapril on survival in patients with reduced left ventricular ejection fractions and congestive heart failure. *New Engl J Med.* 1991;325(5):293–302.

10. GISSI-3 Investigators. GISSI-3: effects of lisinopril and transdermal glyceryl trinitrate singly and together on 6-week mortality and ventricular function after acute myocardial infarction. Gruppo Italiano per lo Studio della Sopravvivenza nell'infarto Miocardico. *Lancet.* 1994;343(8906):1115–1122.

11. The Sixth Report of the Joint National Committee on Prevention, Detection, Evaluation, and Treatment of High Blood Pressure. Available at: http://www.nhlbi.nih.gov/guidelines/hypertension/jncintro.htm.

12. Packer M et al. Double-blind, placebo-controlled study of the effects of carvedilol in patients with moderate to severe heart failure. *Circulation.* 1996;94:2793–2799.

13. Bristow MR et al. Carvedilol produces dose-related improvements in left ventricular function and survival in subjects with chronic heart failure. *Circulation.* 1996;94:2807–2816.

14. Hjalmarson A, Goldstein S, Fagerberg B, Wedel H, Waagstein F, Kjekshus J, et al. Effects of controlled-release metoprolol on total mortality, hospitalizations, and well-being in patients with heart failure: the Metoprolol CR/XL Randomized intervention trial in congestive heart failure (MERIT-HF). MERIT-HF Study Group. *J Am Med Assoc.* 2000;283(10):1295–1302.

15. Packer M et al. Effect of amlodipine on morbidity and mortality in severe chronic heart failure. *New Engl J Med.* 1996;335:1107–1114.

16. Cohn JN, Ziesche S, Smith R, Anand I, Dunkman WB, Loeb H, et al. Effect of the calcium antagonist felodipine as supplementary vasodilator therapy in patients with chronic heart failure treated with enalapril: V-HeFT III. Vasodilator-Heart Failure Trial (V-HeFT) Study Group. *Circulation.* 1997;96(3):856–863.

6 Advanced Heart Failure

Sherry K. Milfred-LaForest

CONTENTS

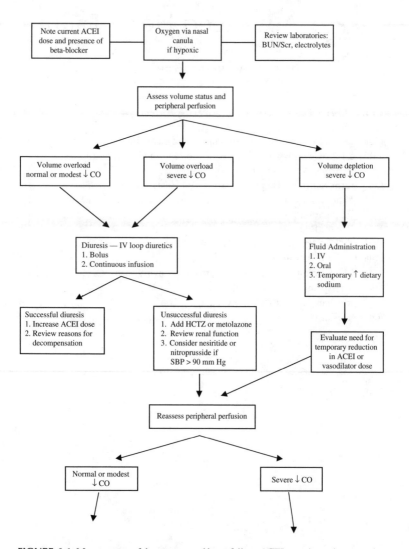

FIGURE 6.1 Management of decompensated heart failure. ACEI = angiotensin converting enzyme inhibitor; BUN = blood urea nitrogen; SCr = serum creatinine; CO = cardiac output; IV = intravenous; HCTZ = hydrochlorothiazide; ARB = angiotensin receptor blocker; BP = blood pressure; PA = pulmonary artery. (Adapted from Pina IL, et al. *J. Am. Coll. Cardiol.* 2001.)

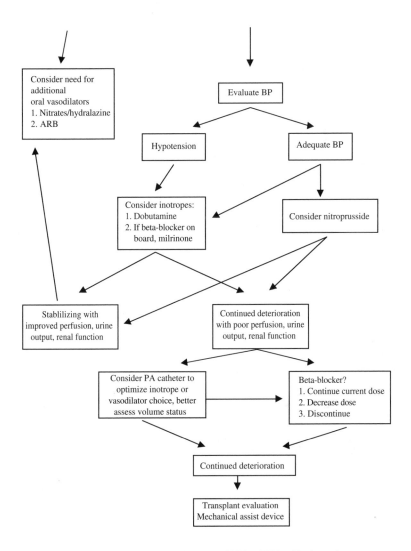

FIGURE 6.1 Continued.

Abbreviations: ACEI — angiotensin converting enzyme inhibitor; BUN — blood urea nitrogen, SCr — serum creatine; CO — cardiac outpu; IV — intravenous; HCTV — hydrochlorothiazide; ARB — angiotensin receptor blocker; BP — blood pressure; PA — pulmonary artery

TABLE 6.1
Hemodynamic Effects of Inotropes and Vasodilators in Advanced Heart Failure[2,3]

Drug	VD	VC	INT	HR	PAP	PCWP	CO	MAP	SVR
Dobutamine	++		++++	↑↑↑	↓↓	↓	↑↑↑	Variable	↓↓
Milrinone	+++		+++	↑↑↑	↓↓↓	↓↓↓	↑↑↑	Variable	↓↓↓
Nesiritide	++++				↓↓↓	↓↓↓	↑	↓↓	↓↓↓↓
Nitroprusside	++++				↓↓↓	↓↓↓	↑	↓↓	↓↓↓↓
Nitroglycerin	+++				↓↓	↓↓	↑ especially if ischemia present	↓↓ especially with volume depletion	↓
Dopamine	+ low dose	+	+++	↑↑↑	↑	↑	↑	↑	↑
Norepinephrine		++++	+	↑↑	↑↑	↑↑	Variable	↑↑↑	↑↑↑
Epinephrine	+ low dose	+++	+++	↑↑↑	↑	↑	↑	↑↑	↑↑
Vasopressin		+++			↑↑	↑		↑↑	↑↑

Abbreviations: VD = vasodilator; VC = vasoconstrictor; INT = inotrope; HR = heart rate; PAP = pulmonary artery pressures; PCWP = pulmonary capillary wedge pressure; CO = cardiac output; MAP = mean arterial pressure; SVR = systemic vascular resistance.

Source: Adapted from Sypniewski E. In: *Pharmacotherapy: A Pathophysiologic Approach.* 3rd ed. DiPiro JT, et al. eds. New York: McGraw-Hill; 1997, 522. With permission.

LONG-TERM INOTROPIC THERAPY IN ADVANCED HEART FAILURE[4,5]

Author's Note: The use of chronic inotropic therapy in heart failure remains controversial. No clinical trial has yet demonstrated a benefit of this therapy on mortality; in fact, small trials have suggested a deleterious effect on mortality due to proarrhythmic effects and increased myocardial oxygen demand of these agents. The data supporting these therapies come largely from small trials or case series and involve benefits in patient quality of life, and potentially decreased hospitalizations and therefore costs. Nevertheless, this therapy is frequently used as a bridge to transplantation for appropriate candidates (inpatient or outpatient) and may be considered as destination therapy for patients in whom no other alternative therapies exist for symptomatic improvement.

PATIENT SELECTION

- Advanced heart failure not amenable to percutaneous coronary or surgical interventions
- Continued heart failure symptoms, volume overload, and/or poor peripheral perfusion despite maximally tolerated doses of appropriate oral pharmacotherapy (e.g., ACE inhibitors, beta-blockers, digoxin, diuretics as needed, other oral vasodilators)*
- Invasive hemodynamic studies performed within 6 months prior to inotrope initiation documenting cardiac index 2.2 l/min/m² and/or pulmonary capillary wedge pressure >20 mm Hg*
- Clinical symptom and/or end organ perfusion improvement with inotropic infusion*
- Documented 20% increase in cardiac index or 20% decrease in pulmonary capillary wedge pressure with inotropic infusion*
- Failed attempt to wean inotropic agent (continuous infusion)*
- Repeated hospitalizations for heart failure (intermittent infusion)*
- Placement of appropriate intravenous access device for long-term infusion therapy
- Adequate resources and support to manage intravenous access in the home (with home care assistance)
- Adequate resources and/or insurance coverage to pay for cost of home care and drug therapy for long-term care

---

* Required for Medicare reimbursement of therapy.

PREPARATION FOR DISCHARGE**

- Clinically significant or life-threatening arrhythmias controlled*
- Patient/caregiver should possess a scale and a home blood pressure–monitoring device
- Home infusion therapy company contacted and accepts patient for service
- Training of patient and caregiver on infusion device — usually a portable infusion pump (e.g., CADD® pump)
- Discussion of advance directive and resuscitation status

PATIENT EDUCATION

- Understanding of end-stage nature of disease and purpose of inotropic therapy
- Daily weights, use of home blood pressure–monitoring device, ability to take apical pulse (or read from blood pressure monitoring device)
- Regular follow-up care with home care nurse and managing cardiologist — electrolytes, renal function, arrhythmias, clinical status
- Other concomitant medications, dietary restrictions, etc.

** Patients who are listed as candidates for heart transplantation may remain as inpatients or be discharged as outpatients depending on clinical status.

TABLE 6.2
Chronic Inotropic Therapy[4,5]

Drug	Usual Doses	Medicare Reimbursment	Monitoring Parameters	Advantages	Disadvantages
Dobutamine Continuous infusion	2–7.5 µg/kg/min 2.5–10 µg/kg/min[a]	80% of costs if criteria[b] met	Electrolytes, renal function, HR, BP, SOB, exercise tolerance, catheter/pump function	Improved quality of life May decrease readmissions for HF, and cost	Tachyphylaxis, increased myocardial oxygen demand, may worsen mortality
Dobutamine Intermittent infusion	2–8 µg/kg/min infusion 4–48 h per week 2.5–10 µg/kg/min at least 1 day per week[a]	80% of costs if criteria[b] met	Electrolytes, renal function, HR, BP, SOB, exercise tolerance, catheter/pump function	Improved quality of life May decrease readmissions for HF, and cost	Increased myocardial oxygen demand, may worsen mortality, some trials have shown no benefit in hospitalization or costs
Milrinone Continuous infusion	0.2–0.5 µg/kg/min 0.375–0.75 µg/kg/min[a]	80% of costs if criteria[b] met	Electrolytes, renal function, HR, BP, SOB, exercise tolerance, catheter/pump function	Improved quality of life May decrease readmissions for HF, and cost. May be used in patients who are receiving beta-blockers	Increased myocardial oxygen demand, may worsen mortality, may have higher out-of-pocket costs to patient

TABLE 6.2 (CONTINUED)
Chronic Inotropic Therapy[4,5]

Drug	Usual Doses	Medicare Reimbursment	Monitoring Parameters	Advantages	Disadvantages
Milrinone Intermittent infusion	0.2–0.5 µg/kg/min 4–72 h per week 0.375–0.75 µg/kg/min at least 1 day per week[a]	80% of costs if criteria[b] met	Electrolytes, renal function, HR, BP, SOB, exercise tolerance, catheter/pump function	Improved quality of life May decrease readmissions for HF, and cost. May be used in patients who are receiving beta-blockers	Increased myocardial oxygen demand, may worsen mortality, may have higher out-of-pocket costs to patient

[a] Doses required for Medicare reimbursement of therapy.
[b] Refer to criteria in "Long-Term Inotropic Therapy in Advanced Heart Failure."
HR = heart rate; BP = blood pressure; SOB = shortness of breath; HF = heart failure.

FOLLOW-UP FOR ADVANCED HEART FAILURE

Maintaining Patients in the Outpatient Environment

Clinic Visits

- Within 2 to 4 weeks of hospital discharge and as clinically indicated
- Signs and symptoms of heart failure
- Vital signs, weight trends, laboratory parameters
  - Electrolytes
  - Renal function
- Uptitration of ACE inhibitors, oral vasodilators, beta-blockers to goal or maximally tolerated doses (see Tables 5.2–5.5)
- Patient/care provider education
  - Diet, sodium restriction, fluid intake
  - Disease state
  - Exercise
- Medication understanding, access, and adherence

Telephone Contacts

- Weight trends
- Diuretic and electrolyte management
- Tolerability of medication changes
- Ongoing education

Chronic Inotropic Therapy

- Considered for patients as a bridge to transplantation or destination therapy
- Has not been shown to improve, and may worsen, mortality; however, heart failure symptoms may be improved
- Home care provider — insurance authorization/payment
- Long-term vascular access catheter for continuous or intermittent infusion
- Ability to teach patient/caregiver regarding catheter care, infusion instructions, managing drug therapy at home
- Routine follow-up with clinic appointments, telephone contacts
- Discussion of advance directives

Transplant Evaluation[6]

Common Indications for Transplant

- Ischemic, dilated, valvular, or congenital cardiomyopathy
- Peak oxygen consumption test (VO_2 max) <14 ml/kg/min or <50% of predicted value for age, size, and gender, and major limitation of patient's daily activities
- Recurrent unstable ischemia not amenable to coronary artery bypass or angioplasty
- Instability of fluid balance and/or renal function not resulting from patient noncompliance with regimen of weight monitoring, flexible use of diuretics, and appropriate oral heart failure medications
- Refractory heart failure symptoms (Class III to IV) in spite of goal or maximally tolerated doses of accepted oral heart failure pharmacotherapy (Tables 5.2–5.5).
- Absence of recent malignant process

Mechanical Assist Devices[7,8]

Bridge to Transplantation or Recovery

- Not currently approved as destination therapy; therefore, patients must be candidates for relatively short-term support, or be an appropriate candidate for transplant
- Devices usually indicated for short-term support (i.e., bridge to recovery)
  - Intra-aortic balloon counterpulsation
  - Extracorporeal nonpulsatile (e.g., centrifugal flow pumps, extracorporeal membrane oxygenation, ECMO)
  - Extracorporeal pulsatile (e.g., Thoratec Ventricular Assist Device; Thoratec Laboratories Corp., ABIOMED BVS 5000®, ABIOMED Cardiovascular, Inc.)
- Devices with potential long-term use (i.e., bridge to transplant)
  - Implantable pulsatile (e.g., Novacor® LVAS, Worldheart Corp. HeartMate® Left Ventricular Assist Device; Thoratec Laboratories Corp.)

Selection Criteria

- Acute catastrophic cardiac event, or inability to wean from cardiopulmonary bypass
- Patients who become clinically unstable while awaiting cardiac transplantation without irreversible end-organ dysfunction
- Absence of irreversible major neurological deficits
- Absence of severe obstructive or restrictive pulmonary disease
- Absence of irreversible coagulopathy
- Body surface area >1.5 m^2 preferable for implantable devices

Anticoagulation

- Intra-aortic balloon counterpulsation: dextran 20 ml/h (postoperatively); heparin with goal aPTT 1.5 to 2.0 × control
- Centrifugal flow pumps: heparin with goal aPTT 40 to 60 seconds, ACT approximately 150 seconds*
- ECMO Venoarterial cannulation (V-A mode): Heparin with goal ACT 180 to 220 seconds
- ECMO Venovenous cannulation (V-V mode): May be managed without systemic anticoagulation, although low-dose heparin is usually employed
- ABIOMED BVS: Heparin with goal aPTT 1.5 to 2.0 × control
- Thoratec Ventricular Assist Device: Heparin with goal aPTT 1.5 to 2.0 × control, Warfarin with goal INR 2.0 to 3.0
- HeartMate LVAD: Aspirin 81 to 325 mg daily or equivalent antiplatelet therapy
- Novacor LVAS: Antiplatelet therapy initiated during perioperative period, heparin with goal aPTT 1.5 × control, Warfarin with goal INR 2.0 to 3.0

Abbreviations

ECMO = extracorporeal membrane oxygenation; ACT = activated clotting time; aPTT = activated partial thromboplastin time; LVAD = left ventricular assist device; LVAS = left ventricular assist system; INR = international normalized ratio.

---

* Center-specific protocol for goal ranges of anticoagulation.

REFERENCES

1. Pina IL et al. Evolving management of decompensated advanced heart failure. *J Am Coll Cardiol*. 2001 (Submitted).
2. Collucci WS. Nesiritide for the treatment of decompensated heart failure. *J Cardiac Failure*. 2001;7:92-100.
3. Sypniewski E. Hypovolemic and cardiogenic shock (Table 23.3). In: *Pharmacotherapy: A Pathophysiologic Approach*. 3rd ed. DiPiro JT, Talbert RL, et al. eds. New York: McGraw-Hill; 1997;522–523.
4. Monk-Tutor M, Powers T. Home care. In: *Pharmacotherapy Self-Assessment Program* 4th ed. *Sites of Care*. St. Louis, MO: American College of Clinical Pharmacy; 2001;257–279.
5. McClosky WW. Use of intravenous inotropic therapy in the home. *Am J Health Syst Pharm*. 1998;55:930–935.
6. Stevenson LW. Medical management before cardiac transplantation. In: *Handbook of Cardiac Transplantation*. Emery RW, Miller LW, eds. Philadelphia: Hanley and Belfus, Inc.; 1996;1–9.
7. Goldstein DJ, Oz ME, Rose EA. Implantable left ventricular assist devices. *N Engl J Med*. 1998;339(21):1522–1533.
8. Goldstein DJ, Oz ME. *Cardiac Assist Devices*. Armonk, NY: Futura Publishing Company, 2000.

7 Post-Cardiac Transplantation

Sherry K. Milfred-LaForest

CONTENTS

TABLE 7.1
Immunosuppression for Chronic Therapy Following Heart Transplantation

Drug	Dosing	Dosing End Point	Maximum Dose	Half-Life	Adverse Effects
		Calcineurin Inhibitors			
Cyclosporine Sandimmune, Neoral, Gengraf,[a] generics[a] 25, 100 mg caps; 100 mg/ml oral solution[b]; 250 mg/5 ml IV vial	3–8 mg/kg/day, usually divided q 12 h IV: po conversion 1:3	Dose varies significantly depending on time from transplant, concomitant drugs Usual goal troughs from 100–350 ng/ml Goal levels may be reduced for toxicity management	Depends on goal levels and assay methodology	10–15 h	CNS toxicity (tremors, headache), renal toxicity, hyperkalemia, hypomagnesemia, hypertension, hyperlipidemia, GI distress, gingival hyperplasia, hirsutism, hyperglycemia, hepatotoxicity, hyperuricemia/gout
Tacrolimus Prograf 0.5, 1, 5 mg caps; 5 mg/ml IV amps	0.1–0.3 mg/kg/day usually divided q 12 h IV: po conversion 1:3 or 1:4	Dose varies significantly depending on time from transplant, concomitant drugs Usual goal troughs from 5–20 ng/ml Goal levels may be reduced for toxicity management	Depends on goal levels and assay methodology	12 h	CNS toxicity (tremors, headache), renal toxicity, hyperkalemia, hypomagnesemia, GI distress, hyperglycemia, hepatotoxicity, hyperuricemia/gout, alopecia, rare hypertension, hyperlipidemia

Antiproliferatives

Drug	Dose		Goal	Half-life	Toxicity
Azathioprine Imuran, generics 50 mg tabs; 100 mg IV vial	1–3 mg/kg daily IV: po conversion 1:2	3 mg/kg/day	Maintain WBC >3000 cells/mm³, platelets >50,000 cells/mm³	5 h (active metabolites)	Myelosuppression, hepatotoxicity, pancreatitis, nausea, vomiting, diarrhea
Mycophenolate Mofetil CellCept 250 mg caps, 500 mg tabs; 200 mg/ml oral suspension; 500 mg IV vial	2000–3000 mg/day, divided bid	Depends on tolerability and trough levels (if monitored by transplant center)	Maintain WBC >3000 cells/mm³, platelets >50,000 cells/mm³ Mycophenolic acid levels may be monitored, with varying methods and assays Usual goal for trough levels 2–4 ng/ml	16–18 h (mycophenolic acid)	Nausea, vomiting, diarrhea, anorexia, myelosuppression
Cyclophosphamide Cytoxan 50 mg tabs	1 mg/kg daily	Not defined	Maintain WBC >3000 cells/mm³, platelets >50,000 cells/mm³ Lower doses may be used if combined with other antiproliferatives	7.5 h	Myelosuppression, nausea, vomiting, diarrhea, stomatitis, blurred vision, rare hepatotoxicity or hemorrhagic cystitis
Methotrexate Rheumatrex 2.5 mg tabs	2.5–10 mg twice weekly	10 mg twice weekly depending on tolerability and rejection response	Maintain WBC >3000 cells/mm³, platelets >50,000 cells/mm³	2–8 h	Nausea, vomiting, diarrhea, stomatitis, rash, alopecia, hepatotoxicity, rare pulmonary toxicity

TABLE 7.1 (CONTINUED)
Immunosuppression for Chronic Therapy Following Heart Transplantation

Drug	Dosing	Dosing End Point	Maximum Dose	Half-Life	Adverse Effects
		mTOR Inhibitors			
Sirolimus Rapamune 1 mg tabs; 1 mg/ml oral solution	Loading dose of 3 × maintenance dose; average maintenance doses vary from 2–5 mg/day	Dose varies significantly depending on time from transplant, concomitant drugs Usual goal troughs from 5–20 ng/ml Goal levels may be reduced for toxicity management	Depends on goal levels and assay methodology; little published data on use in heart transplantation	60 h	Hyperlipidemia, myelosuppression, hypokalemia, hepatotoxicity, diarrhea
		Corticosteroids			
Prednisone Deltasone, Orasone, generics 1, 2.5, 5, 10, 20, 50 mg tabs; 5 mg/5ml oral solution, 5 mg/ml oral solution (intensol)	Variable depending on time from transplant, may start at 1 mg/kg/ day and taper	Some centers using steroid weaning or steroid avoidance protocols with very low doses	Not defined	3.4 h	Pituitary-adrenal axis suppression, fluid retention, electrolyte imbalances, hypertension, hyperlipidemia, hyperglycemia, increased appetite, weight gain, moon

facies, buffalo hump, hirsutism, osteoporosis, mood alterations, thinning skin, acne, proximal muscle weakness, growth retardation (children), cataracts

CNS = central nervous system; GI = gastrointestinal; WBC = white blood cell count.

a AB rated with Neoral.

b Sandimmune and Neoral only.

TABLE 7.2
Immunosuppression for Induction Therapy or Rejection Treatment Following Heart Transplantation

Drug	Dosing	Dosing End Point	Maximum Dose	Half-Life	Adverse Effects
Corticosteroids					
Prednisone Deltasone, Orasone generics 1, 2.5, 5, 10, 20, 50 mg tabs; 5 mg/5ml oral solution, 5 mg/ml oral solution (intensol)	Oral pulses (1–3 mg/kg/day × 3–5 days) may be used to treat mild–moderate rejection	Resolution of rejection	Not defined	3.4 h	Pituitary-adrenal axis suppression, fluid retention, electrolyte imbalances, hypertension, hyperlipidemia, hyperglycemia, increased appetite, weight gain, moon facies, buffalo hump, hirsutism, osteoporosis, mood alterations, thinning skin, acne, proximal muscle weakness, growth retardation (children), cataracts

Methylprednisolone Solu-Medrol, A-Methapred, generics 40, 125, 500, 1000, 2000 mg IV vials	Rejection treated with high-dose pulses (500–1000 mg/day, 15 mg/kg/day × 3–5 days)	Resolution of rejection	Not defined	2 h	Pituitary-adrenal axis suppression, fluid retention, electrolyte imbalances, hypertension, hyperlipidemia, hyperglycemia, increased appetite, mood alterations, proximal muscle weakness

Antibodies

Antithymocyte globulin, Equine Atgam 50 mg/5 ml IV amps	10–15 mg/kg/day Premedication with antihistamine, antipyretic, ± steroid recommended	Resolution of rejection. Allow for minimization of other immuno-suppressants post-transplant or additional therapy for high-risk patients (induction therapy) Maintain WBC >2000 cells/mm^3, platelets >50,000 cells/mm^3	25 mg/kg/day for up to 14 days (manufacturer's maximum recommended dose 20 mg/kg/day)	6 days	Neutropenia, anemia, thrombocytopenia, infusion related reactions (chills, rigors, shortness of breath, malaise, nausea, headache), thrombophlebitis, serum sickness, rare hypersensitivity

TABLE 7.2 (CONTINUED)
Immunosuppression for Induction Therapy or Rejection Treatment Following Heart Transplantation

Drug	Dosing	Dosing End Point	Maximum Dose	Half-Life	Adverse Effects
Antithymocyte globulin Rabbit Thymoglobulin 25 mg IV vial	1–1.5 mg/kg/day Premedication with antihistamine, antipyretic, ± steroid recommended	Resolution of rejection Allow for minimization of other immuno-suppressants post-transplant or additional therapy for high-risk patients (induction therapy) Maintain WBC >2000 cells/mm^3, platelets >50,000 cells/mm^3	2.5 mg/kg/day for up to 14 days (manufacturer's maximum recommended dose 1.5 mg/kg/day)	2–3 days; therapeutic effects may persist 14 days or more following full treatment course	Neutropenia, anemia, thrombocytopenia, infusion-related reactions (chills, rigors, shortness of breath, malaise, nausea, headache), thrombophlebitis, serum sickness, rare hypersensitivity
Orthoclone OKT3 Muromonab CD3 5 mg/5 ml IV amp	5 mg/day Premedication with high-dose steroids, antihistamine, antipyretic recommended	Resolution of rejection Allow for minimization of other immuno-suppressants post-transplant or additional therapy for high-risk patients (induction therapy)	10 mg/day for up to 14 days	Duration of action: 2–5 days	Cytokine release syndrome (fever, chills, rigors, hypotension, tachycardia, shortness of breath, bronchospasm, pulmonary edema),

Drug	Dose	Comments		Half-life / Duration	Adverse effects
Basiliximab Simulect 20 mg IV vial	20 mg on day of transplant and postoperative day 4	Two dose regimen For induction therapy only, not rejection treatment	20 mg	7 days; Duration of action with full course: 36 days	nausea/vomiting/ diarrhea, headache, rare seizures, aseptic meningitis, hypersensitivity, development of anti-murine antibodies
Daclizumab Zenepax 5 mg/5 ml IV vial	1 mg/kg on day of transplant and every 14 days for a total of 5 doses	Five dose regimen For induction therapy only, not rejection treatment	2 mg/kg (manufacturer's maximum recommended dose 1 mg/kg)	20 days; duration of action with full course: 120 days	Nausea, vomiting, headache, dizziness (incidence similar to placebo in clinical trials), rare hypersensitivity
Antiproliferatives					
Cyclophosphamide Cytoxan 50 mg tabs	1 mg/kg daily	Resolution of rejection Maintain WBC >3000 cells/mm^3, platelets >50,000 cells/mm^3	Not defined	7.5 h	Myelosuppression, nausea, vomiting, diarrhea, stomatitis, blurred vision, rare hepatotoxicity or hemorrhagic cystitis

TABLE 7.2 (CONTINUED)
Immunosuppression for Induction Therapy or Rejection Treatment Following Heart Transplantation

Drug	Dosing	Dosing End Point	Maximum Dose	Half-Life	Adverse Effects
Methotrexate Rheumatrex 2.5 mg tabs	2.5–10 mg twice weekly	Resolution of rejection Maintain WBC >3000 cells/mm^3, platelets >50,000 cells/mm^3 Lower doses may be used if combined with other antiproliferatives	10 mg twice weekly depending on tolerability and rejection response	2–8 h	Nausea, vomiting, diarrhea, stomatitis, rash, alopecia, hepatotoxicity, rare pulmonary toxicity

WBC = white blood cell count.

TABLE 7.3
Grading of Cardiac Biopsies for Rejection

	Pathology	Interpretation
Cellular Biopsy Grade		
0	No evidence of lymphocyte infiltration or myocyte damage	No acute rejection
1A	Focal lymphocytic infiltrate without necrosis	Focal, mild acute rejection
1B	Diffuse but sparse lymphocytic infiltrate without necrosis	Diffuse, mild acute rejection
2	Single focus of aggressive lymphocytic infiltrate and/or myocyte damage	Focal, moderate acute rejection
3A	Multifocal aggressive lymphocytic infiltrate and/or myocyte damage	Multifocal moderate acute rejection
3B	Diffuse inflammatory process with necrosis	Diffuse, borderline severe acute rejection
4	Diffuse, aggressive polymorphous infiltrate with necrosis, ± hemorrhage, edema, vasculitis	Severe acute rejection
Immunofluorescence Findings		
Positive direct immuno-fluorescence with complement, with or without interstitial fibrin	Antibody deposition with endothelial cell activation, edema, and hemorrhage	Mild humoral rejection
Positive direct immuno-fluorescence with complement, interstitial fibrin prominent	Antibody deposition with endothelial cell activation, edema, hemorrhage, ± vasculitis	Moderate humoral rejection
Positive direct immunofluorescence with complement, interstitial leakage of fibrin, complement, and immunoglobulin	Antibody deposition with extensive lymphocyte and other cellular infiltrates, myocyte distortion, edema, and hemorrhage	Severe humoral rejection

Source: Adapted from Billingham ME, et al. *J. Heart Lung Transplant.* 1990;9(6):588; Olsen SL et al. *J. Heart Lung Transplant.* 1993: 12(Suppl 1):si36. With permission.

TABLE 7.4
Common Infections in Heart Transplant Recipients[4-6]

Infection	Timing	Prevention	Treatment
Bacterial			
Surgical wound	Within first month	First- or second-generation cephalosporin perioperatively	As determined by culture results
Line infections	Any time indwelling lines present	Meticulous care of central lines	As determined by culture results
Urinary tract	Any time	n/a	As determined by culture results
Pneumonia	Any time	n/a	As determined by culture results
Viral			
Cytomegalovirus (CMV)	Months 1–6, after treatment for rejection, lower risk after 6 months	Ganciclovir, valganciclovir, CMV hyperimmune globulin	Ganciclovir, foscarnet, valganciclovir, CMV hyperimmune globulin (for pulmonary or multi-organ disease)
Herpes simplex (HSV)	Within first 6 months, lower risk after 6 months	Acyclovir (if ganciclovir not used for CMV)	Acyclovir, foscarnet
Varicella zoster (VZV)	Months 1–6, after treatment for rejection, lower risk after 6 months	Acyclovir (if ganciclovir not used for CMV)	acyclovir, foscarnet
Fungal			
Oral candidiasis	Highest first 3 months, after treatment of rejection, lower risk from 3–12 months	Nystatin, clotrimazole troches	Fluconazole

TABLE 7.4 (CONTINUED)
Common Infections in Heart Transplant Recipients[4-6]

Infection	Timing	Prevention	Treatment
Candidemia	First 6 months	n/a	Fluconazole, itraconazole, amphotericin B, amphotericin B lipid formulation
Cryptococcus	Highest first 6 months, lower risk after 6 months	n/a	Fluconazole, amphotericin B, amphotericin B lipid formulation
Aspergillus	Highest first 6 months, lower risk after 6 months	Avoidance of exposure to spores	Amphotericin B, amphotericin B lipid formulation, itraconazole
Other			
Pneumocystis carinii	Months 1–6, after treatment of rejection, lower risk after 6 months	Trimethoprim/sulfa methoxazole, dapsone, pentamidine	Trimethoprim/sulfameth-oxazole, clindamycin + primaquine, pentamidine, atovaquone
Toxoplasmosis	Months 1–6, after treatment of rejection	Trimethoprim/sulfa methoxazole, dapsone, pyrimethamine	Pyrimethamine + sulfadiazine + folinic acid, clindamycin, azithromycin, clarithromycin

n/a = not applicable.

COMMON CARDIOVASCULAR COMPLICATIONS FOLLOWING HEART TRANSPLANTATION

Author's Note: There are no consensus documents from the heart transplant community specifically addressing management of these complications. Rather, center-specific protocols are commonly employed. These will vary based on the immunosuppression regimen used, patient population (i.e., children vs. adults), and experience of the transplant physicians. Provided below are broad guidelines and factors that should be considered in managing heart transplant recipients with these common comorbid conditions.

HYPERTENSION[7,8]

Factors Contributing to Occurrence

- Pretransplant history
- Immunosuppressive therapy
  - Cyclosporine and corticosteroids have been associated with increases in blood pressure. Patients receiving tacrolimus-based immunosuppression have lower incidences of hypertension than those receiving cyclosporine-based regimens.
- Renal insufficiency

Goal Blood Pressure

- Generally follow JNC VI guidelines (see Chapter 1)
- Most centers consider ideal blood pressure to be <140/90 mm Hg

Management Considerations

- Hypertension is often refractory, requiring polypharmacy to control blood pressure adequately. Adverse effects and complexity of drug regimens may be significant factors in pharmacotherapy choices.

Anti-Hypertensive Drug Therapy

- Calcium channel blockers
  - May provide protection against transplant coronary artery disease and/or nephrotoxicity

- Drug interactions to varying degrees with cyclosporine, tacrolimus, and sirolimus; levels of immunosuppressants require careful monitoring as agents are started, titrated, and discontinued
- ACE inhibitors/angiotensin II receptor blockers
  - May provide protection against transplant coronary artery disease
  - May provide protection against cyclosporine nephrotoxicity (controversial)
  - Caution in patients with renal insufficiency (Scr >2.5)
  - Drug interaction with cyclosporine and tacrolimus; potential for additive hyperkalemia requiring careful monitoring of renal function and potassium levels
- Diuretics
  - May be helpful in African American patients in combination with ACE inhibitor or angiotensin receptor blocker
  - Drug interaction with sirolimus; potential for additive hypokalemia
  - May be beneficial in patients with hyperkalemia
  - Caution in patients with renal insufficiency — dehydration may exacerbate cyclosporine or tacrolimus nephrotoxicity
- Alpha-2 adrenergic agonists
  - Caution with bradycardia in denervated heart
  - Adverse effect profile may limit use
- Other vasodilators
  - Caution with excessive orthostasis in denervated heart
  - Caution with minoxidil in combination with cyclosporine due to potentially additive hirsutism
  - Adverse effect profile may limit use
- Beta-blockers
  - Generally poorly tolerated in heart transplant recipients due to denervated heart and altered response of peripheral vasodilatory mechanisms
  - May exacerbate hyperlipidemia or glucose intolerance

Alteration in Immunosuppression

- Patients with refractory hypertension may be candidates for altered immunosuppression
  - Changing from cyclosporine-based to tacrolimus-based immunosuppression
  - Steroid minimization or weaning protocols

HYPERLIPIDEMIA[9,10]

Factors Contributing to Occurrence

- Pretransplant history
- Post-transplant weight gain
- Immunosuppressive therapy
  - Cyclosporine, corticosteroids, and sirolimus have been associated with increases in LDL, total cholesterol, and triglyceride levels. Patients receiving tacrolimus-based immunosuppression have lower incidences of dyslipidemia than those receiving cyclosporine-based regimens.

Goal Lipid Levels

- Optimal goal lipid levels for heart transplant recipients not defined. Consider risk of transplant coronary vasculopathy (see below). Patients with ischemic etiology for transplant, other vascular disease, diabetes, or documented allograft vasculopathy require aggressive therapy (i.e., goal LDL <100).

Management Considerations

Nonpharmacologic Therapy

- Weight control
- Dietary modification: decrease total cholesterol and saturated fat intake (see Chapter 2)
- Moderate physical activity (once cleared from surgical standpoint) — consider cardiac rehabilitation program

Lipid Lowering Drug Therapy

- HMG CoA reductase inhibitors (Statins)
  - Pravastatin and simvastatin shown to have beneficial effect on transplant coronary artery disease and mortality
  - Concern for drug interactions with cyclosporine (tacrolimus, sirolimus possible as well)
  - Increased levels of statin can lead to myositis, rhabdomyolysis

- Risk highest for statins with greatest dependence on cytochrome P450 3A4 system for metabolism (e.g., simvastatin, lovastatin)
- Consider monitoring of creatine kinase levels in patients at high risk for myopathy
- Maximum recommended doses of statins in patients on cyclosporine:
  Atorvastatin 10–20 mg/day
  Fluvastatin 40–80 mg/day
  Lovastatin 20 mg/day
  Pravastatin 20–40 mg/day
  Simvastatin 10–20 mg/day
    Lower doses are manufacturer's recommendations; higher doses have been used safely in clinical trials
- Bile acid-binding resins
  - Drug interaction potential with immunosuppressants
  - Decreased absorption of lipid-soluble drugs (e.g., cyclosporine, tacrolimus, sirolimus) requiring separation of doses by at least 4 h
  - Decreased absorption of drugs undergoing enterohepatic recirculation (e.g., mycophenolate mofetil) such that combination should be avoided if possible
  - Timing requires increased complexity of drug regimens, which may decrease adherence
- Nicotinic acid
  - Effective in mixed dyslipidemia, which is common in heart transplant population
  - Often poorly tolerated in patients with glucose intolerance
  - Combination therapy with statins may increase risk of myositis in presence of cyclosporine or other immunosuppressants
- Fibric acid derivatives
  - Effective against hypertriglyceridemia, but little effect on LDL
  - Combination therapy with statins may increase risk of myositis in presence of cyclosporine or other immunosuppressants

Alteration in Immunosuppression

- Patients with refractory dyslipidemias may be candidates for altered immunosuppression:
  - Changing from cyclosporine or sirolimus-based to tacrolimus-based immunosuppression
  - Steroid minimization or weaning protocols

TRANSPLANT CORONARY ARTERY VASCULOPATHY[11,12]

Characteristics

- Diffuse, distal locations in coronary arteries
- Concentric intimal (smooth muscle) proliferation
- Develops over period of months to years

Factors Contributing to Occurrence

- Older donor age
- Donor hypertension
- Donor or recipient male sex
- African American recipient
- Recipient hypertension
- Recipient hyperlipidemia
- Recipient diabetes/insulin resistance
- Smoking
- Cytomegalovirus infection
- Prolonged ischemic time at the time of transplantation
- Rejection
- Decreased levels of antithrombin III and microvascular deposition of fibrin in allograft in early post-transplant period

Diagnosis and Monitoring

- Coronary angiography
- Intravascular coronary ultrasound
- Noninvasive methods for detection of ischemia
  - Dobutamine echocardiography

Management Considerations

Invasive Management

- Evaluate for presence of traditional atherosclerotic lesions in combination with transplant coronary artery vasculopathy
- Revascularization
  - Not usually amenable to angioplasty, stenting, or bypass
  - May be possible if discrete lesions identified

Pharmacologic Therapy

- ACE inhibitors may decrease intimal proliferation and slow progression of disease
- HMG CoA reductase inhibitors (pravastatin, simvastatin) may decrease intimal proliferation and slow progression of disease
- Calcium channel blockers (diltiazem) may slow progression of disease
- Antiplatelet therapy (aspirin) may slow progression of disease (controversial)
- Treatment of hypertension, hyperlipidemia, diabetes
- Modification and/or augmentation of immunosuppression
  - Mycophenolate mofetil-based regimens have slower progression of disease than azathioprine-based regimens
- Treatment of signs of ischemia or heart failure

Retransplantation

- Only definitive "cure" for transplant coronary artery disease; however, candidate status, survival rate, and ethical considerations affect suitability of this option on a patient-by-patient basis

FOLLOW-UP MONITORING AFTER HEART TRANSPLANTATION

Author's Note: The information provided below represents broad guidelines and factors that should be considered in managing heart transplant recipients. Center-specific protocols commonly employed will vary based on the immunosuppression regimen used, patient population (i.e., children vs. adults), and experience of the transplant physicians.

REJECTION/TRANSPLANT CORONARY ARTERY VASCULOPATHY

- Regular cardiac biopsies during first 6 to 12 months, then on an "as-needed" or protocol basis
- Echocardiography at least annually or if indicated by symptoms
- Evaluation of coronary arteries and/or presence of ischemia at least annually or if indicated

INFECTION

- Daily assessment of temperature and any symptoms of illness
- Aggressive evaluation of fever, symptoms of illness when noted
- Patient education regarding procedures to avoid infection (e.g., hand-washing)
- Regular assessment of white blood cell count during first 6–12 months
- Monitoring of viral titers or antigens
  - Cytomegalovirus
  - Epstein-Barr virus (children)
- Annual influenza vaccination, pneumococcal vaccination prior to transplant and every 6 years

DRUG TOXICITY

- Daily assessment of vital signs, weight
  - Regular assessment of laboratory parameters
  - Electrolytes
  - Renal function
  - Complete blood count
  - Liver function
  - Lipid profile
- Regular assessment of immunosuppressive medication levels
  - Cyclosporine
  - Tacrolimus
  - Sirolimus
  - Mycophenolate mofetil (mycophenolic acid) in some centers
- Monitoring of blood glucose
  - At least every 6 months in patients without diabetes
  - As indicated in patients with diabetes along with hemoglobin A1c
  - Treatment as needed with glucose-lowering agents (caution with metformin due to increased likelihood of renal dysfunction with calcineurin inhibitors)
- Pretransplant assessment of osteoporosis risk and regular monitoring for fractures and/or bone density status
  - Consider use of calcium supplementation, calcitonin, and/or bisphosphonates in high-risk patients or patients with evidence of fractures

- Assessment of other patient-specific adverse effects
  - Headache or neuropathy
  - Gastrointestinal upset or diarrhea
  - Gout
  - Cosmetic effects (hirsutism, gingival hyperplasia), which may have impact on drug adherence

MALIGNANCY

- Use of sunscreen and avoidance of tobacco products and other known carcinogens
- Regular skin evaluation for suspicious lesions or moles
- Mammography and gynecological, or prostate evaluation as recommended by American Cancer Society
- Evaluation of gastrointestinal tract via colonoscopy or flexible sigmoidoscopy as recommended by American Cancer Society
- Radiographic imaging of chest at least annually

PATIENT EDUCATION

- Daily vital signs
  - Heart rate, blood pressure, temperature, weight
- Signs and symptoms of rejection
- Preparations for and procedure of cardiac biopsy
- Infection prevention and surveillance measures
- Activity
  - Lifting (weight limitations)
  - Driving
  - Exercise (consider cardiac rehab program)
- Medication regimen
- Dietary recommendations
  - Low fat, low cholesterol
  - Low potassium (if needed)
  - Diabetic diet (if needed)
  - Sodium restriction (if needed)
- Corresponding with donor families
- When to call transplant center

REFERENCES

1. Billingham ME et al. A working formulation for the standardization of nomenclature in the diagnosis of heart and lung rejection: heart rejection study group (Table 1). *J Heart Lung Transplant.* 1990;9(6): 587–593.

2. Olsen SL et al. Vascular rejection in heart transplantation: clinical correlation, treatment options, and future considerations (Table 1). *J Heart Lung Transplant.* 1993;12(2 suppl 1):s135–142.

3. Fishman JA, Rubin RH. Infection in organ transplant recipients. *New Engl J Med.* 1998;338(24):1741–1751.

4. Love KR. Prevention and prophylaxis of infection in thoracic transplantation. In: *Handbook of Cardiac Transplantation.* Emery RW, Miller LW, eds. Philadelphia: Hanley and Belfus, Inc., 1996;17–30.

5. Green MR, Olyaei AJ. Infectious complications in transplant recipients. In: *Pharmacotherapy Self-Assessment Program.* 4th ed. *Infectious Diseases.* St. Louis, MO: American College of Clinical Pharmacy; 2001;87–106.

6. Ventura HO et al. Cyclosporine-induced hypertension in cardiac transplantation. *Med Clin North Am.* 1997;81(6):1347–1357.

7. Midtvedt K, Neumayer HH. Management strategies for posttransplant hypertension. *Transplantation.* 2000;70(11 suppl):ss64–69.

8. Lake KD. Management of post-transplant obesity and hyperlipidemia. In: *Handbook of Cardiac Transplantation.* Emery RW, Miller LW, eds. Philadelphia: Hanley and Belfus, Inc., 1996;147–164.

9. Ballantyne CM et al. Treatment of hyperlipidemia after heart transplantation and rationale for the Heart Transplant Lipid Registry. *Am J Cardiol.* 1996;78(5):532–535.

10. Costanzo MR et al. Heart transplant coronary artery disease detected by coronary angiography: a multiinstitutional study of preoperative donor and recipient risk factors. *J Heart Lung Transplant.* 1998;17(8):744–753.

11. Aranda JM, Hill J. Cardiac transplant vasculopathy. *Chest.* 2000;118(6): 1792–1800.

8 Atrial Arrhythmias

Cynthia A. Sanoski

CONTENTS

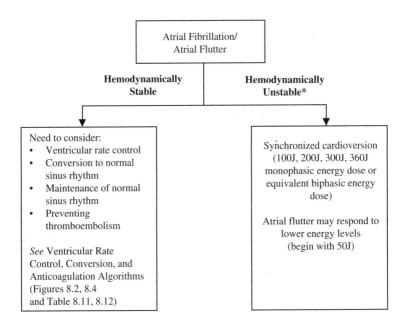

FIGURE 8.1 General acute treatment algorithm for atrial fibrillation/atrial flutter. *Defined as patients with acute myocardial infarction, symptomatic hypotension, ventricular rate >150 bpm, or acute heart failure. J = joules. (Adapted from The American Heart Association in Collaboration with the International Liaison Committee on Resuscitation. *Circulation*. 2000; 102(Suppl I): I-158–I-165.)

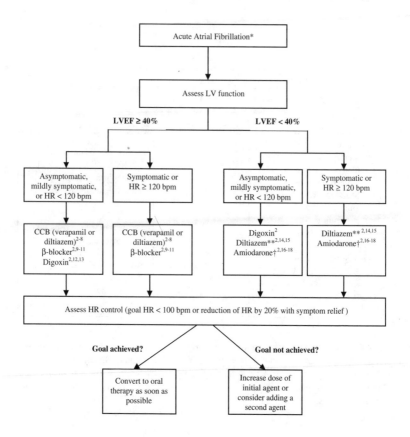

FIGURE 8.2 Algorithm for acute ventricular rate control in atrial fibrillation. *All drugs in this algorithm should be administered intravenously. **Do not use IV diltiazem for more than 24 h in patients with left ventricular dysfunction. †Because of its ability to convert AF/AFl to normal sinus rhythm, IV amiodarone should be reserved for use within the first 48 h of arrhythmia onset. In patients with AF/AFl for more than 48 h, IV amiodarone should only be used for those who have been adequately anticoagulated. LV = left ventricle, LVEF = left ventricular ejection fraction; HR = heart rate; bpm = beats per minute; CCB = calcium channel blocker; IV = intravenous; AF/AFl = atrial fibrillation/atrial flutter. (Adapted from The American Heart Association in Collaboration with the International Liaison Committee on Resuscitation. *Circulation.* 2000; 102(Suppl I): I-158–I-165.)

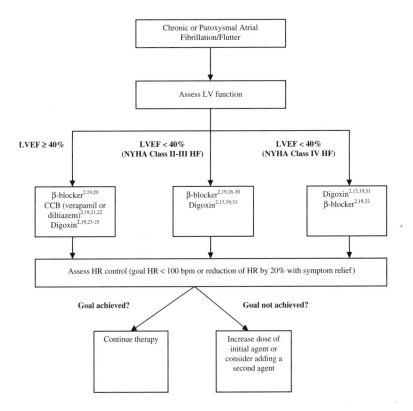

FIGURE 8.3 Algorithm for ventricular rate control in chronic or paroxysmal atrial fibrillation/flutter. LV = left ventricle; LVEF = left ventricular ejection fraction; NYHA = New York Heart Association; HF = heart failure; CCB = calcium channel blocker; HR = heart rate; bpm = beats per minute. (Adapted from Tisdale JE, Moser JL. In: Mueller BA, et al., eds. *Pharmacotherapy Self-Assessment*, 4th ed. Kansas City, MO: ACCP; 2001.)

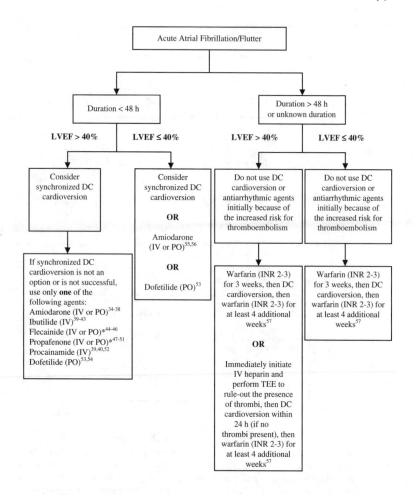

FIGURE 8.4 Algorithm for conversion of hemodynamically stable atrial fibrillation/flutter to normal sinus rhythm. *IV flecainide and IV propafenone are not available in the United States. LVEF = left ventricular ejection fraction; DC = direct current; IV = intravenous; PO = oral; INR = International Normalized Ratio; TEE = transesophageal echo-cardiogram. (Adapted from The American Heart Association in Collaboration with the International Liaison Committee on Resuscitation. *Circulation.* 2000; 102(Suppl I): I-158–I-165 and Fuster, V et al. *J Am Coll Cardiol.* 2001; 38:1231.)

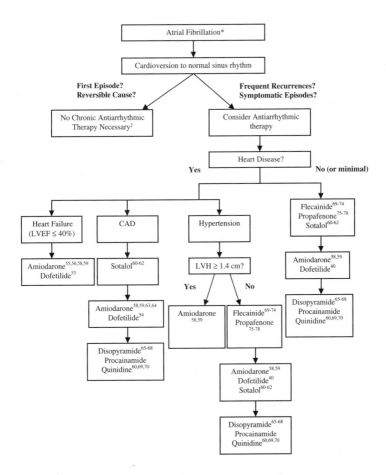

FIGURE 8.5 Algorithm for maintenance of normal sinus rhythm following cardioversion of atrial fibrillation. LVEF = left ventricular ejection fraction; CAD = coronary artery disease; LVH = left ventricular hypertrophy; *Drugs are listed alphabetically and not in order of suggested use. (Adapted from Fuster V, et al. *J Am Coll Cardiol.* 2001;38:1231.)

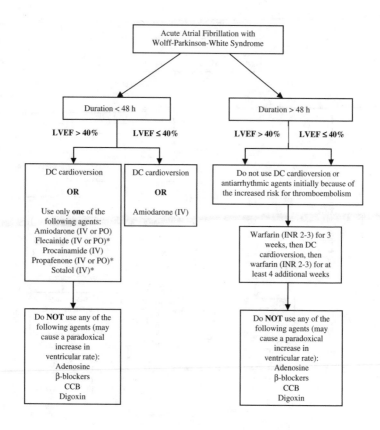

FIGURE 8.6 Algorithm for acute ventricular rate control and conversion to normal sinus rhythm in hemodynamically stable atrial fibrillation with Wolff-Parkinson-White syndrome. *IV flecainide, IV propafenone, and IV sotalol are not available in the United States. LVEF = left ventricular ejection fraction; DC = direct current; IV = intravenous; PO = oral; CCB = calcium channel blocker; INR = International Normalized Ratio. (Adapted from The American Heart Association in Collaboration with the International Liaison Committee on Resuscitation. *Circulation*. 2000; 102(Suppl I): I-158–I-165.)

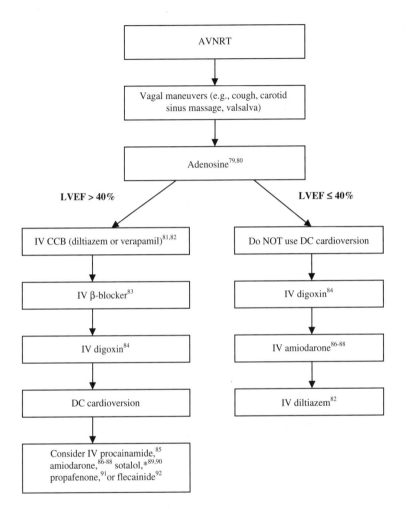

FIGURE 8.7 Algorithm for maintenance of hemodynamically stable acute atrioventricular nodal reentrant tachycardia. AVNRT = atrioventricular nodal reentrant tachycardia; LVEF = left ventricular ejection fraction; IV = intravenous; CCB = calcium channel blocker; DC = direct current; *IV flecainide, IV propafenone, and IV sotalol are not available in the U.S. (Adapted from The American Heart Association in Collaboration with the International Liaison Committee on Resuscitation. *Circulation.* 2000; 102(Suppl I): I-158–I-165.)

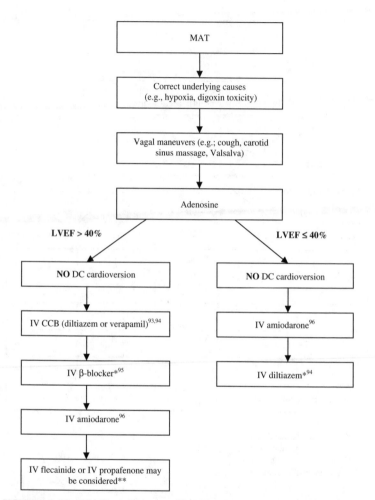

FIGURE 8.8 Algorithm for maintenance of hemodynamically stable acute multifocal atrial tachycardia. MAT = multifocal atrial tachycardia; LVEF = left ventricular ejection fraction; DC = direct current; IV = intravenous; CCB = calcium channel blocker. *Digoxin may also be used for rate control (ineffective in terminating MAT). However, this agent should only be used if digoxin toxicity has been ruled out as the cause of the MAT. **IV flecainide and IV propafenone are not available in the U.S. (Adapted from The American Heart Association in Collaboration with the International Liaison Committee on Resuscitation. *Circulation.* 2000; 102(Suppl I): I-158–I-165.)

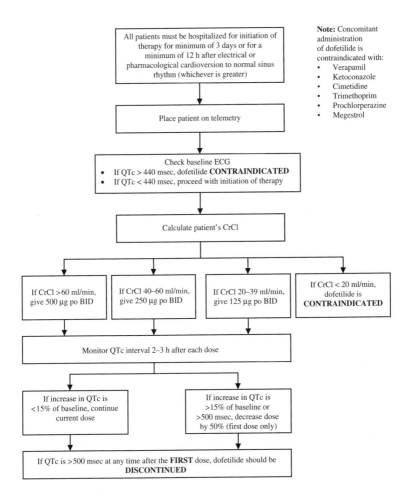

FIGURE 8.9 Dofetilide dosing and monitoring algorithm. ECG = electrocardiogram; QTc = corrected QT interval; CrCl = creatinine clearance; BID = twice daily.

TABLE 8.1
Class Ia Antiarrhythmics

Drug	Half-Life	Route of Elimination	Usual Dose	Maximum Dose	Therapeutic Range	Adverse Effects	Monitoring Parameters	Ref.
Disopyramide	4–10 h	Hepatic/renal	<50 kg: IR: 100 mg po q 6 h CR: 200 mg po q 12 h >50 kg: IR: 150 mg po q 6 h CR: 300 mg po q 12 h Renal insufficiency (only use IR form): CrCl 30–40 ml/min: 100 mg po q 8 h CrCl 15–30 ml/min: 100 mg po q 12 h CrCl < 15 ml/min: 100 mg po q 24 h	<50 kg: 400 mg/day >50 kg: 800 mg/day	2–5 μg/ml	Nausea, anorexia, dry mouth, urinary retention, blurred vision, constipation, heart failure exacerbation, torsades de pointes, hypotension	ECG (QTc interval, QRS duration), BP, signs/ symptoms of heart failure, electrolytes (K^+, Mg^{2+})	97, 98

| Procainamide | PA: 2.5–5 h[a] NAPA: 6–8 h | Hepatic/renal PA: ~15–30% is eliminated renally as unchanged drug; remainder is metabolized in liver to NAPA NAPA: Renally eliminated | IV: LD: 15–17 mg/kg over 25–60 min MD: 1–4 mg/min continuous infusion PO: Usual dose: 50 mg/kg/day IR: 250–500 mg q 3–6 h Procan SR®: 500–1000 mg q 6 h Procanbid®: 500–2000 mg q 12 h Use with caution, if at all, in renal insufficiency | Should be adjusted for each patient individually based upon renal function, plasma levels, and therapeutic response | PA: 4–10 µg/ml NAPA: 15–25 µg/ml Total: 10–30 µg/ml | Diarrhea, nausea, vomiting, SLE-like syndrome (rash, arthralgias, fever, pericarditis, pleuritis), torsades de pointes, hypotension (with IV), agranulocytosis | ECG (QTc interval, QRS duration), BP, PA/NAPA levels, CBC with differential, electrolytes (K^+, Mg^{2+}) | 97, 99–101 |

TABLE 8.1 (CONTINUED)
Class Ia Antiarrhythmics

Drug	Half-Life	Route of Elimination	Usual Dose	Maximum Dose	Therapeutic Range	Adverse Effects	Monitoring Parameters	Ref.
Quinidine	6–8 h	Hepatic	Quinidine sulfate: 200–400 mg po q 6 h Quinidine gluconate: 324 mg po q 8–12 h	Quinidine sulfate: 600 mg po q 6 h Quinidine gluconate: 972 mg po q 8–12 h	2–5 µg/ml	Torsades de pointes, diarrhea, stomach cramps, nausea, vomiting, hypotension, thrombo-cytopenia, fever, cinchonism (tinnitus, blurred vision, headache)	ECG (QTc interval, QRS duration), BP, quinidine levels, CBC, liver function tests, electrolytes (K^+, Mg^{2+})	102, 103

[a] PA half-life also depends on acetylator phenotype (fast vs. slow).

IR = immediate release; CR = controlled release; CrCl = creatinine clearance; ECG = electrocardiogram; QTc interval = corrected QT interval; BP = blood pressure; K^+ = potassium; Mg^{2+} = magnesium; PA = procainamide; NAPA = N-acetyl procainamide; IV = intravenous; LD = loading dose; MD = maintenance dose; PO = oral; SR = sustained release; SLE = systemic lupus erythematosus; CBC = complete blood count.

TABLE 8.2
Class Ic Antiarrhythmics

Drug	Half-Life	Route of Elimination	Usual Dose	Maximum Dose	Therapeutic Range	Adverse Effects	Monitoring Parameters	Ref.
Flecainide	7–22 h	Hepatic/renal	LD (for cardioversion): 200–300 mg po × 1 dose MD: Initial dose, 50 mg po q 12 h; increase in 50-mg increments q 12 h every 4–7 days, until desired response	150 mg po every 12 h	Not monitored clinically	Dizziness, visual disturbances, dyspnea, headache, tremor, nausea, heart failure exacerbation, ventricular tachycardia	ECG (QRS duration), baseline echocardiogram (to evaluate left ventricular function)	104–107
Propafenone	Extensive metabolizers (90% of patients): 2–8 h Poor metabolizers (10% of patients): 10–32 h	Hepatic	LD (for cardioversion): 450–600 mg po × 1 dose MD: 150 mg po every 8 h	300 mg po every 8 h	Not monitored clinically	Bradycardia, AV block, heart failure exacerbation, ventricular tachycardia, nausea, vomiting, dizziness, fatigue, bronchospasm, headache, taste disturbances	ECG (QRS duration, PR interval), HR, BP, baseline echocardiogram (to evaluate left ventricular function)	108, 109

LD = loading dose; MD = maintenance dose; ECG = electrocardiogram; AV = atrioventricular; HR = heart rate; BP = blood pressure.

TABLE 8.3
Class II Antiarrhythmics

Drug	Half-Life	Route of Elimination	Usual Dose	Maximum Dose	Therapeutic Range	Adverse Effects	Monitoring Parameters	Ref.
Esmolol	9 min	In blood by esterases	500 µg/kg IV bolus over 1 min, then start 50 µg/kg/min infusion for 4 min; if inadequate response, rebolus with 500 µg/kg IV over 1 min and increase infusion by 50 µg/kg/min; repeat this process until desired response achieved or maximum dose of 300 µg/kg/min is reached; when discontinuing therapy, can decrease infusion rate by 25–50 µg/kg/min every 5–10 min	300 µg/kg/min	Not monitored clinically	Hypotension, bradycardia, heart block, heart failure exacerbation, bronchospasm, dizziness, drowsiness, nausea, phlebitis	ECG (PR interval), HR, BP	2, 110

| Metoprolol | 3–4 h | Hepatic | IV: 2.5–5 mg over 2 min; can repeat every 2 min up to a total of 3 doses PO: IR: Initial dose: 25 mg bid Initial dose: 6.25 mg bid (in patients with NYHA FC II-III heart failure) | PO: IR: 450 mg/day; 200 mg/day (in patients with heart failure) | Not monitored clinically | Hypotension, bradycardia, heart block, drowsiness, fatigue, heart failure exacerbation, depression, nausea, vomiting, bronchospasm, cold extremities | ECG (PR interval), HR, BP, RR, weight | 2 |
| | | | SR (Metoprolol CR/XL®): Initial dose: 50 mg qd; Initial dose: 12.5 mg qd (in patients with NYHA FC II-III heart failure) Titrate dose to desired response (HR <100 bpm) | SR: 400 mg/day; 200 mg/day (in patients with heart failure) | | | | |

TABLE 8.3 (CONTINUED)
Class II Antiarrhythmics

Drug	Half-Life	Route of Elimination	Usual Dose	Maximum Dose	Therapeutic Range	Adverse Effects	Monitoring Parameters	Ref.
Propranolol	4–6 h	Hepatic	IV: 1 mg over 1 min; may repeat every 5 min up to total dose of 5 mg PO: Initial dose: 10–20 mg q 6–8 h; titrate dose to desired response (HR <100 bpm); usual dose: 80–240 mg/day in 2–4 divided doses	IV: Maximum total dose: 0.15 mg/kg PO: 480 mg/day	Not monitored clinically	Hypotension, bradycardia, heart block, depression, nightmares, insomnia, fatigue, lethargy, heart failure exacerbation, bronchospasm, cold extremities	ECG (PR interval), HR, BP, RR, weight	2

ECG = electrocardiogram; HR = heart rate; BP = blood pressure; IV = intravenous; PO = oral; IR = immediate release; bid = twice daily; NYHA = New York Heart Association; FC = functional class; SR = sustained release; qd = every day; bpm= beats per minute; RR = respiratory rate.

TABLE 8.4
Class III Antiarrhythmics

Drug	Half-Life	Route of Elimination	Usual Dose	Maximum Dose	Therapeutic Range	Adverse Effects	Monitoring Parameters	Ref.
Amiodarone	40–55 days (range = 25–107 days)	Hepatic	IV: See Table 8.7 PO: See Table 8.7	LD should be given until patient has received ~10 g; the dose can then be tapered to the MD regimen	1–2 mg/l (serum levels have not been shown to correlate with clinical efficacy)	IV: Hypotension, bradycardia, heart block, phlebitis PO: Hypothyroidism, hyperthyroidism, pulmonary fibrosis, bradycardia, heart block, corneal microdeposits, optic neuritis, nausea, vomiting, anorexia, constipation, LFTs, hepatitis, tremor, ataxia, paresthesias, photosensitivity, blue-gray skin discoloration, insomnia	ECG (QTc interval, QRS duration, PR interval), HR, BP, CXR, PFTs, TFTs, LFTs, ophthalmologic exam (see Table 8.8 for monitoring guidelines)	2, 111– 115

TABLE 8.4 (CONTINUED)
Class III Antiarrhythmics

Drug	Half-Life	Route of Elimination	Usual Dose	Maximum Dose	Therapeutic Range	Adverse Effects	Monitoring Parameters	Ref.
Dofetilide	8–10 h	Renal/ hepatic	Initial dose: 500 μg po bid; dose must be adjusted in patients with renal insufficiency (see Figure 8.9); dose must also be adjusted based on QTc interval (see Figure 8.9)	Dose should be based upon renal function; prescribers have the option of using a dose lower than what is recommended for a certain renal function; however, prescribers should not use doses higher than recommended for a patient's renal fuention	Not monitored clinically	Torsades de pointes, headache, dizziness, insomnia, chest pain, nausea, diarrhea, dyspnea, respiratory tract infection	ECG (QTc interval), renal function, electrolytes (K^+, Mg^{2+})	116, 117

Ibutilide	2–12 h	Hepatic	<60 kg: 0.01 mg/kg IV over 10 min ≥60 kg: 1 mg IV over 10 min If AF/AFl does not terminate within 10 min after end of initial infusion, can give a second dose (as above) over 10 min	No more than two doses should be administered	Not monitored clinically	Torsades de pointes, headache, nausea	ECG (QTc interval), electrolytes (K^+, Mg^{2+})	118, 119

TABLE 8.4 (CONTINUED)
Class III Antiarrhythmics

Drug	Half-Life	Route of Elimination	Usual Dose	Maximum Dose	Therapeutic Range	Adverse Effects	Monitoring Parameters	Ref.
Sotalol	12 h	Renal	Initial dose: 80 mg po bid; dose can be increased at 3-day intervals to maximum of 160 mg po bid	160 mg po bid	Not monitored clinically	Torsades de pointes, bradycardia, chest pain, palpitations, fatigue, dizziness, lightheadedness, weakness, dyspnea, bronchospasm, heart failure exacerbation, nausea, vomiting, diarrhea	ECG (QTc interval, PR interval), HR, electrolytes (K^+, Mg^{2+})	120, 121

Dosing interval must be adjusted in patients with renal insufficiency: CrCl 40–60 ml/min: every 24 h; CrCl <40 ml/min: contra-indicated

IV = intravenous; PO = oral; LD = loading dose; MD = maintenance dose; LFTs = liver function tests; ECG = electrocardiogram; QTc interval = corrected QT interval; HR = heart rate; BP = blood pressure; CXR = chest x-ray; PFTs = pulmonary function tests; TFTs = thyroid function tests; bid = twice daily; CrCl = creatinine clearance; K^+ = potassium; Mg^{2+} = magnesium; AF = atrial fibrillation; AFl = atrial flutter.

TABLE 8.5
Class IV Antiarrhythmics

Drug	Half-Life	Route of Elimination	Usual Dose	Maximum Dose	Therapeutic Range	Adverse Effects	Monitoring Parameters	Ref.
Diltiazem	4–6 h	Hepatic	IV: LD: 0.25 mg/kg ABW over 2 min; if response inadequate after 15 min, can repeat with 0.35 mg/kg ABW over 2 min Continuous infusion: 5–15 mg/h PO: IR: Initial dose: 30 mg qid SR (Cardizem CD®): Initial dose: 120 mg qd; titrate dose to desired response (HR <100 bpm); usual dose: 120–360 mg/day	IV: Maximum infusion rate: 15 mg/h PO: 480 mg/day	Not monitored clinically	Hypotension, bradycardia, heart block, headache, flushing, dizziness, edema, heart failure exacerbation	ECG (PR interval), HR, BP, weight	2, 122

| Verapamil | 2–8 h | Hepatic | IV:
LD: 2.5–5 mg over 2 min; if response inadequate after 15–30 min, can double initial dose and administer over 2 min
Continuous Infusion:
5–10 mg/h
PO:
IR: Initial dose: 80 mg tid
SR: Initial dose: 240 mg qd
Titrate dose to desired response (HR <100 bpm); Usual dose: 240–360 mg/day | IV:
Maximum infusion rate: 15 mg/h
PO: 480 mg/day | Not monitored clinically | Hypotension, bradycardia, heart block, heart failure exacerbation, headache, flushing, dizziness, edema, constipation | ECG (PR interval), HR, BP, weight | 2, 123, 124 |

IV = intravenous; LD = loading dose; ABW = actual body weight; po = oral; HR = heart rate; bpm = beats per minute; ECG = electrocardiogram; HR = heart rate; BP = blood pressure; tid = three times daily.

TABLE 8.6
Other Antiarrhythmics

Drug	Half-life	Route of Elimination	Usual Dose	Maximum Dose	Therapeutic Range	Adverse Effects	Monitoring Parameters	Ref.
Adenosine	<10 s	Metabolized in the blood	6 mg IV push; if not effective within 1–2 min, can give 12 mg IV push; may give another 12 mg IV push, if needed in 1–2 min; each dose should be followed with 10–20 ml normal saline flush	Maximum single dose: 12 mg	Not monitored clinically	Flushing, palpitations, chest pain, dyspnea, headache (all are brief in duration)	ECG, HR, BP	125

| Digoxin | 26–48 h | Renal/hepatic | LD:
IV: 10–15 µg/kg IBW (give 50% of LD initially, then give 25% of LD 6 h later, then give remaining 25% of LD 6 h later

PO: 10–15 µg/kg IBW (same administration guidelines as IV, but must adjust dose for difference in bioavailability) (bioavailability of tablets ~80%)

MD:
IV: 0.125–0.25 mg qd
PO: 0.125–0.5 mg qd | Maintenance dose may be calculated by using the following equation:
$MD = TBS * \% DL$
where
$TBS = 10\text{–}15$ µg/kg IBW
$\% DL = 14 + (CrCl/5)$ | 0.8–2 ng/ml; serum concentrations should be obtained at least 6 h after an oral dose and 4 h after an IV dose | Heart block, AV junctional tachycardia, atrial tachycardia with block, ventricular arrhythmias, visual disturbances (blurred vision, yellow/green halos), headache, dizziness, weakness, nausea, vomiting, anorexia, diarrhea Digoxin immune Fab can be used to treat severe or life-threatening digoxin toxicity (Table 8.10) | ECG (PR interval), HR, renal function, signs/symptoms of toxicity, electrolytes (K^+, Mg^{2+}, Ca^{2+}), digoxin levels (especially when compliance is questioned, renal function declines, or toxicity is suspected) | 126–128 |

IV = intravenous; ECG = electrocardiogram; HR = heart rate; BP = blood pressure; LD = loading dose; IBW = ideal body weight; MD = maintenance dose; qd = every day; po = oral; TBS = total body stores; % DL = percent daily loss; CrCl = creatinine clearance; AV = atrioventricular; K^+ = potassium; Mg^{2+} = magnesium; Ca^{2+} = calcium.

TABLE 8.7
Amiodarone Dosing for Atrial Fibrillation

Intravenous Amiodarone

Loading dose	5–7 mg/kg administered over 30–60 min
Maintenance dose	1200–1800 mg/day given via continuous infusion; convert patient to oral therapy when hemodynamically stable and able to take oral medications

Oral Amiodarone

Loading dose	800–1200 mg/day in 2–3 divided doses for 1 week, until patient receives ~10 g total, then give MD; loading doses should be administered with food to minimize gastrointestinal symptoms
Maintenance dose	200 mg po QD (it may be possible to maintain some patients on doses as low as 100 mg/day)

Guidelines for Converting from IV to Oral Therapy

Duration of IV Amiodarone Infusion	Initial Daily Dose of Oral Amiodarone
<1 week	800–1200 mg[a]
1–3 weeks	400 mg[a]
>3 weeks	200 mg

MD = maintenance dose; po = oral; qd = every day; IV = intravenous.

[a] These daily doses should be continued until the patient receives ~10 g total load. Patient can then be given MD.

TABLE 8.8
Amiodarone Monitoring Guidelines[a]

Monitoring Parameter	Monitoring Frequency
Chest x-ray	Baseline and then every 12 months
Thyroid function tests	Baseline and then every 6 months
Liver function tests	Baseline and then every 6 months
Pulmonary function tests	Baseline and then on an as-needed basis if patient becomes symptomatic or if chest x-ray is abnormal
Ophthalmologic exam	Baseline and then every 12 months
Electrocardiogram	Baseline and then with every visit

[a] If clinically necessary, more frequent monitoring may become warranted.

Source: Adapted from Goldschlager N, et al. *Arch Intern Med.* 2000;160:1741.

TABLE 8.9
Major Amiodarone Drug Interactions

Drug	Interaction	Intervention
Warfarin[129-134]	Amiodarone potentiates the anticoagulant effects of Warfarin	Reduce the dose of Warfarin by approximately 40 or 30% when using a maintenance amiodarone dose of 400 or 200 mg/day, respectively; monitor INR closely; monitor for bleeding
Digoxin[135]	Amiodarone may double digoxin levels	Consider reducing the digoxin dose by 50%; monitor digoxin levels closely; monitor for signs/symptoms of digoxin toxicity
Cyclosporine[136]	Amiodarone may increase cyclosporine levels	Monitor cyclosporine levels closely and adjust the cyclosporine dose accordingly; monitor for signs/symptoms of cyclosporine toxicity
β-blockers, diltiazem, verapamil	Concomitant therapy may result in additive bradycardia and/or AV block	Monitor HR and ECG (PR intervals) closely
Phenytoin[137]	Amiodarone may increase phenytoin levels; phenytoin may decrease amiodarone levels	Monitor phenytoin levels closely; monitor for signs/symptoms of phenytoin toxicity; monitor ECG for arrhythmia recurrence
Other QT-prolonging drugs	Concomitant therapy may excessively prolong the QT interval	Monitor QTc interval closely; if QTc >440 msec, patient may be at risk for torsades de pointes
Procainamide[138]	Amiodarone may increase procainamide and NAPA levels	Consider reducing procainamide dose by 25% and monitoring procainamide and NAPA levels closely; monitor QTc interval closely (patient may be at risk for torsades de pointes); if possible, may want to avoid concomitant use

TABLE 8.9 (CONTINUED)
Major Amiodarone Drug Interactions

Drug	Interaction	Intervention
Quinidine[139]	Amiodarone may increase quinidine levels	Monitor quinidine levels closely; monitor QTc interval closely (patient may be at risk for torsades de pointes); if possible, may want to avoid concomitant use
Lidocaine[140,141]	Amiodarone may increase lidocaine levels	Monitor lidocaine levels closely (especially after 24 h of use); if possible, may want to avoid concomitant use

INR = international normalized ratio; AV = atrioventricular; HR = heart rate; ECG = electrocardiogram; QTc = corrected QT interval; NAPA = *N*-acetyl procainamide.

TABLE 8.10
Digoxin Immune Fab (Digibind®, DigiFab®) Dosing and Monitoring Guidelines

Indications

- Life-threatening arrhythmias secondary to digoxin
- Acute digoxin ingestion (>10 mg in adults, >4 mg in children, or serum digoxin level >10 ng/ml)
- Hyperkalemia (serum potassium >5 mEq/l) in setting of digoxin toxicity

Dosing Guidelines

Each vial of Digibind®, or DigiFab®, (40 mg) will bind 0.5 mg of digoxin

The dose of either of these agents can be based on:

- Serum digoxin level:

$$\text{Number of vials} = \frac{\text{Digoxin level (ng/ml) * weight (kg)}}{100}$$

- Total amount of digoxin ingested:

Number of 0.25 mg tabs Ingested[a]	Number of Vials	Dose of Digibind®/DigiFab® (mg)
5	2	80
10	4	160
25	10	400
50	20	800
75	30	1200
100	40	1600
150	60	2400
200	80	3200

- If the serum digoxin level or total amount of digoxin is not known:

Acute toxicity → Use 10 vials of Digibind® or DigiFab®
Chronic toxicity → Use 5 vials of Digibind® or DigiFab®

TABLE 8.10 (CONTINUED)
Digoxin Immune Fab (Digibind®, DigiFab®) Dosing and Monitoring Guidelines

Administration

- Reconstitute each vial with 4 ml of sterile water, which results in concentration of 10 mg/ml
- This reconstituted solution can be further diluted in normal saline to final concentration of 1 mg/ml.
- Administer infusion over 30 min

Monitoring

- A serum digoxin level should be obtained prior to administration of Digibind®, or DigiFab®; this level may be difficult to evaluate if 6–8 h have not elapsed since the last dose of digoxin
- After Digibind®/DigiFab® therapy, serum digoxin levels will significantly increase and will not be an accurate representation of digoxin body stores; digoxin levels may not become accurate until the Digibind/DigiFab is eliminated from the body (half-life 15–20 h; longer in patients with renal insufficiency)
- Monitor potassium concentrations closely after Digibind® or DigiFab®, administration as hypokalemia may develop
- Monitor the ECG for development or recurrence of life-threatening arrhythmias

ECG = electrocardiogram.

[a] 0.25 mg tablets are 80% bioavailable.

TABLE 8.11
Risk Stratification for Thromboembolism in Patients with Atrial Fibrillation

Risk Stratification
High-risk factors:
  Prior stroke, transient ischemic attack, or systemic embolus
  History of hypertension
  Poor left ventricular systolic function
  Age >75 years
  Rheumatic mital valve disease
  Prosthetic heart valve
Moderate-risk factors:
  Age = 65–75 years
  Diabetes mellitus
  Coronary artery disease with normal left ventricular systolic function

High-risk patient: ≥1 high-risk factor, or >1 moderate-risk factor

Moderate-risk patient: Only 1 moderate-risk factor

Low-risk patient: *NO* high-risk or moderate-risk factors

Source: Adapted from Albers GW, et al. *Chest*. 2001;119:1945.

TABLE 8.12
Recommendations for Antithrombotic Therapy in Atrial Fibrillation

Risk Category	Antithrombotic Regimen
High-risk	Warfarin (target INR 2.5; range = 2.0–3.0)
High-risk patient with contraindication to Warfarin or unwilling to take Warfarin	Aspirin 325 mg po qd can be used as alternative to Warfarin therapy
Moderate-risk	Warfarin (target INR 2.5; range = 2.0–3.0) **OR** Aspirin 325 mg po qd Need to select therapy based upon ability to monitor Warfarin therapy, patient's risk of bleeding, and patient preference
Low-risk	Aspirin 325 mg po qd

INR = international normalized ratio; qd = every day.

Source: Adapted from Albers GW, et al. *Chest*. 2001;119:1945.

TABLE 8.13

Recommendations for Antithrombotic Therapy for Elective Cardioversion of Atrial Fibrillation or Atrial Flutter

Arrhythmia	Antithrombotic Regimen
Atrial fibrillation or atrial flutter (<48 h in duration)[a]	Initiate IV heparin upon presentation; may proceed with DC cardioversion *without* 3-week period of precardioversion Warfarin therapy[a]
Atrial fibrillation or atrial flutter (>48 h in duration)	Warfarin (target INR 2.5; range = 2.0–3.0) for 3 weeks before and at least 4 weeks following cardioversion
If TEE to be performed	Initiate IV heparin and perform TEE to exclude presence of thrombi; DC cardioversion can then be performed within 24 h if no thrombi detected; Warfarin (target INR 2.5; range = 2.0–3.0) should be continued for at least 4 weeks following cardioversion; if thrombi are detected on TEE, patient will require Warfarin (target INR 2.5; range = 2.0–3.0) for 3 weeks before and at least 4 weeks following cardioversion

IV = intravenous; DC = direct current; INR = international normalized ratio; TEE = transesophageal echocardiogram.

[a] For patients with a previous history of stroke/thromboembolism, or severe left ventricular systolic dysfunction, clinicians should consider performing a TEE or anticoagulating the patient for 3 weeks prior to DC cardioversion, as these patients may be at increased risk for thromboembolism.

Source: Adapted from Albers GW, et al. *Chest*. 2001;119:1945.

TABLE 8.14
Follow-Up Plans for Atrial Arrhythmias

Heart rate and blood pressure should be monitored periodically
- Heart rate goal <100 beats per minute
- Patients who are hospitalized for initiation of ventricular rate control and/or antiarrhythmic therapy should be on telemetry so that heart rate and rhythm can be continually monitored

12-lead electrocardiogram should be performed periodically
- Assess for recurrent arrhythmia
- Measure QRS duration (for Type Ia/Ic antiarrhythmics and amiodarone), QTc interval (for Type Ia and III antiarrhythmics), and PR interval (for Type I, II, III, and IV antiarrhythmics)

If patient is on Warfarin therapy, INR should be monitored every week for the first month (until patient has consistently remained in the therapeutic range), and then every month for as long as the patient continues on the drug (should be monitored more frequently if interacting medication is initiated)
- Evaluate patient for any signs/symptoms of bleeding
- Instruct patient to contact physician or pharmacist immediately if he or she experiences any unusual or excessive bleeding
- Reinforce importance of dietary compliance (i.e., to eat consistent quantities of vitamin K containing foods), medication compliance, and INR monitoring
- Instruct patient to contact his or her pharmacist when taking any new prescription, over-the-counter, or herbal therapies.

Assess patient for drug-induced adverse effects
- See Tables 8.1 to 8.6

Monitor all patients on amiodarone therapy for adverse effects on a regular basis
- See Table 8.8 for monitoring guidelines
- Educate patient on signs/symptoms of adverse effects associated with amiodarone

Routine monitoring of digoxin levels is not necessary in patients with atrial fibrillation; a digoxin level can be obtained when the following conditions apply:
- Renal function deteriorates
- Compliance is questioned
- Toxicity is suspected
- Concomitant therapy with an interacting drug is initiated

Plasma amiodarone and/or desethylamiodarone concentrations do not need to be monitored as there does not appear to be a relationship between these concentrations and the clinical efficacy of the drug

Screen and appropriately monitor patients for any drug interactions

REFERENCES

1. The American Heart Association in Collaboration with the International Liaison Committee on Resuscitation (ILCOR). Guidelines 2000 for Cardiopulmonary Resuscitation and Emergency Cardiovascular Care: An International Consensus on Science. *Circulation* 2000;102(Suppl I):I-158–I-165.

2. Fuster V et al. ACC/AHA/ESC guidelines for the management of patients with atrial fibrillation: a report of the American College of Cardiology/American Heart Association Task Force on Practice Guidelines and the European Society of Cardiology Committee for Practice Guidelines and Policy Conferences. *J Am Coll Cardiol.* 2001;38:1231–1266.

3. Tommaso C et al. Atrial fibrillation and flutter: immediate control and conversion with intravenously administered verapamil. *Arch Intern Med.* 1983;143:877–881.

4. Phillips BG et al. Comparison of intravenous diltiazem and verapamil for the acute treatment of atrial fibrillation and atrial flutter. *Pharmacotherapy.* 1997;17:1238–1245.

5. Hwang MH et al. Double-blind crosover randomized trial of intravenously administered verapamil: its use for atrial fibrillation and flutter following open heart surgery. *Arch Intern Med.* 1984;144:491–494.

6. Tisdale JE et al. A randomized, double-blind comparison of intravenous diltiazem and digoxin for atrial fibrillation after coronary artery bypass surgery. *Am Heart J.* 1998;135:739–747.

7. Schreck DM, Rivera AR, Tricarico VJ. Emergency management of atrial fibrillation and flutter: intravenous diltiazem versus intravenous digoxin. *Ann Emerg Med.* 1997;29:135–140.

8. Ellenbogen KA et al. Safety and efficacy of intravenous diltiazem in atrial fibrillation or atrial flutter. *Am J Cardiol.* 1995;75:45–49.

9. Gray RJ et al. Esmolol: a new ultrashort-acting beta-adrenergic blocking agent for rapid control of heart rate in postoperative supraventricular tachyarrhythmias. *J Am Coll Cardiol.* 1985;5:1451–1456.

10. Amsterdam EA, Kulcyski J, Ridgeway MG. Efficacy of cardioselective beta-adrenergic blockade with intravenously administered metoprolol in the treatment of supraventricular tachyarrhythmias. *J Clin Pharmacol.* 1991;31:714–718.

11. Rehnqvist N. Clinical experience with intravenous metoprolol in supraventricular tachyarrhythmias: a multicentre study. *Ann Clin Res.* 1981;13(suppl 30):68–72.

12. Falk RH et al. Digoxin for converting recent-onset atrial fibrillation to sinus rhythm: a randomized double-blinded trial. *Ann Intern Med.* 1987;106:503–506.

13. Roberts SA et al. Effectiveness and costs of digoxin for atrial fibrillation and flutter. *Am J Cardiol.* 1993;72:567–573.

14. Goldenberg IF et al. Intravenous diltiazem for the treatment of patients with atrial fibrillation or flutter and moderate to severe congestive heart failure. *Am J Cardiol.* 1994;74:884–889.

15. Heywood JT et al. Effects of intravenous diltiazem on rapid atrial fibrillation accompanied by congestive heart failure. *Am J Cardiol.* 1991;67:1150–1152.

16. Cotter G et al. Conversion of recent onset paroxysmal atrial fibrillation to normal sinus rhythm: the effect of no treatment and high-dose amiodarone: a randomized, placebo-controlled study. *Eur Heart J*. 1999;20:1833–1842.

17. Galve E et al. Intravenous amiodarone in treatment of recent-onset atrial fibrillation: results of a randomized, controlled study. *J Am Coll Cardiol*. 1996;27:1079–1082.

18. Clemo HF et al. Intravenous amiodarone for acute heart rate control in the critically ill patient with atrial tachyarrhythmias. *Am J Cardiol*. 1998;81:594–598.

19. Segal JB et al. The evidence regarding the drugs used for ventricular rate control. *J Fam Pract*. 2000;49:47–59.

20. Atwood JE et al. Effects of beta-adrenergic blockade on exercise performance in patients with chronic atrial fibrillation. *J Am Coll Cardiol*. 1987;10:314–320.

21. Lundstrom T, Ryden L. Ventricular rate control and exercise performance in chronic atrial fibrillation: effects of diltiazem and verapamil. *J Am Coll Cardiol*. 1990;16:86–90.

22. Lang R et al. Verapamil improves exercise capacity in chronic atrial fibrillation: double-blind crossover study. *Am Heart J*. 1983;105:820–824.

23. Jordaens L. Conversion of atrial fibrillation to sinus rhythm and rate-control by digoxin in comparison to placebo. *Eur Heart J*. 1997;18:643–648.

24. Blumgart H. The reaction to exercise of the heart affected by auricular fibrillation. *Heart*. 1924;11:49–56.

25. Falk RH, Leavitt JI. Digoxin for atrial fibrillation: a drug whose time has gone *Ann Intern Med*. 1991;114:573–575.

26. Packer M et al. The effect of carvedilol on morbidity and mortality in patients with chronic heart failure. *New Engl J Med*. 1996;334:1349–1355.

27. CIBIS II Investigators and Committees. The Cardiac Insufficiency Bisoprolol Study II (CIBIS-II): a randomized trial. *Lancet*. 1999;353:9–13.

28. MERIT-HF Study Group. Effect of metoprolol CR/XL in chronic heart failure: Metoprolol CR/XL Randomized Intervention Trial in Congestive Heart Failure (MERIT-HF). *Lancet*. 1999;353:2001–2007.

29. Heart Failure Society of America. HFSA guidelines for management of patients with heart failure caused by left ventricular dysfunction: pharmacological approaches. *J Cardiac Failure*. 1999;5:357–382.

30. Hunt SA et al. ACC/AHA guidelines for the evaluation and management of chronic heart failure in the adult: executive summary. A report of the American College of Cardiology/American Heart Association Task Force on Practice Guidelines. *J Am Coll Cardiol*. 2001;38:2101–2113.

31. The Digitalis Investigators Group. The effect of digoxin on mortality and morbidity in patients with heart failure. *New Engl J Med*. 1997;336:525–533.

32. Packer M et al., for the Carvedilol Prospective Randomized Cumulative Survival Study Group. Effect of carvedilol on survival in severe chronic heart failure. *New Engl J Med*. 2001;344:1651–1658.

33. Tisdale JE, Moser JL. Tachyarrhythmias. In: Mueller BA, Bertch KE, Dunsworth TS, eds. *Pharmacotherapy Self-Assessment Program*, 4th ed. Kansas City, MO: ACCP; 2001.

34. Galve E et al. Intravenous amiodarone in treatment of recent-onset atrial fibril-
    lation: results of a randomized, controlled study. *J Am Coll Cardiol.*
    1996;27:1079–1082.

35. Kerin NZ, Faitel K, Naini M. The efficacy of intravenous amiodarone for the
    conversion of chronic atrial fibrillation: amiodarone vs. quinidine for conversion
    of atrial fibrillation. *Arch Intern Med.* 1996;156:49–53.

36. Hou ZY et al. Acute treatment of recent-onset atrial fibrillation and flutter with
    a tailored dosing regimen of intravenous amiodarone: a randomized, digoxin-
    controlled study. *Eur Heart J.* 1995;16:521–528.

37. Noc M, Stajer D, Horvat M. Intravenous amiodarone versus verapamil for acute
    conversion of paroxysmal atrial fibrillation to sinus rhythm. *Am J Cardiol.*
    1990;65:679–680

38. Vardas PE et al. Amiodarone as a first-choice drug for restoring sinus rhythm in
    patients with atrial fibrillation: a randomized, controlled study. *Chest.*
    2000;117:1538–1545.

39. Stambler BS, Wood MA, Ellenbogen KA. Antiarrhythmic actions of intravenous
    ibutilide compared with procainamide during human atrial flutter and fibrillation:
    electrophysiologic determinants of enhanced conversion efficacy. *Circulation.*
    1997;96:4298–4306.

40. Volgman AS et al. Conversion efficacy and safety of intravenous ibutilide com-
    pared with intravenous procainamide in patients with atrial flutter or fibrillation.
    J Am Coll Cardiol. 1998;31:1414–1419.

41. Vos MA et al., for the Ibutilide/Sotalol Comparator Study Group. Superiority of
    ibutilide (a new class III agent) over dl-sotalol in converting atrial flutter and
    atrial fibrillation. *Heart.* 1998;79:568–575.

42. Stambler BS et al., for the Ibutilide Repeat Dose Study Investigators. Efficacy
    and safety of repeated intravenous doses of ibutilide for rapid conversion of atrial
    flutter or fibrillation. *Circulation.* 1996;94:1613–1621.

43. Ellenbogen KA et al. Efficacy of intravenous ibutilide for rapid termination of
    atrial fibrillation and atrial flutter: a dose-response study. *J Am Coll Cardiol.*
    1996;28:130–136.

44. Borgear A et al. Flecainide versus quinidine for conversion of atrial fibrillation
    to sinus rhythm. *Am J Cardiol.* 1986;58:496–498.

45. Suttorp MJ et al. Intravenous flecainide versus verapamil for acute conversion
    of paroxysmal atrial fibrillation or flutter to sinus rhythm. *Am J Cardiol.*
    1989;63:693–696.

46. Capucci A et al. Effectiveness of loading oral flecainide for converting recent-
    onset atrial fibrillation to sinus rhythm in patients without organic heart disease
    or with only systemic hypertension. *Am J Cardiol.* 1992;70:69–72.

47. Capucci A et al. A controlled study on oral propafenone versus digoxin plus
    quinidine in converting recent onset atrial fibrillation to sinus rhythm. *Int J
    Cardiol.* 1994;43:305–313.

48. Azpitarte J et al. Value of single oral loading dose of propafenone in converting
    recent-onset atrial fibrillation: results of a randomized, double-blind, controlled
    study. *Eur Heart J.* 1997;18:1649–1654.

49. Botto GL et al. Conversion of recent onset atrial fibrillation to sinus rhythm using a single oral loading dose of propafenone: comparison of two regimens. *Int J Cardiol.* 1997;58:55–61.

50. Boriani G et al. Propafenone for conversion of recent-onset atrial fibrillation: a controlled comparison between oral loading dose and intravenous administration. *Chest.* 1995;108;355–358.

51. Boriani G et al. Oral propafenone to convert recent-onset atrial fibrillation in patients with and without underlying heart disease: a randomized, controlled trial. *Ann Intern Med.* 1997;126:621–625.

52. Madrid AH et al. Comparison of flecainide and procainamide in cardioversion of atrial fibrillation. *Eur Heart J.* 1993;14:1127–1131.

53. Torp-Pedersen C et al., for the Danish Investigations of Arrhythmia and Mortality on Dofetilide Study Group. Dofetilide in patients with congestive heart failure and left ventricular dysfunction. *New Engl J Med.* 1999;341:857–865.

54. Singh S et al. Efficacy and safety of oral dofetilide in converting to and maintaining sinus rhythm in patients with chronic atrial fibrillation or atrial flutter: the Symptomatic Atrial Fibrillation Investigative Research on Dofetilide (SAFIRE-D) study. *Circulation.* 2000;102:2385–2390.

55. Doval HC et al., for Grupo de Estudio de la Sobrevida en la Insuficiencia Cardiaca en Argentina (GESICA). Randomized trial of low-dose amiodarone in severe congestive heart failure. *Lancet.* 1994;344:493–498.

56. Singh SN et al. Amiodarone in patients with congestive heart failure and asymptomatic ventricular arrhythmia: survival trial of antiarrhythmic Therapy in congestive heart failure (CHF-STAT). *New Engl J Med.* 1995;333:77–82.

57. Albers GW et al. Antithrombotic therapy in atrial fibrillation. *Chest.* 2001;119:194S–206S.

58. Roy D et al., for the Canadian Trial of Atrial Fibrillation Investigators. Amiodarone to prevent recurrence of atrial fibrillation. *New Engl J Med.* 2000;342:913–920.

59. Kochiadakis GE et al. Low dose amiodarone and sotalol in the treatment of recurrent, symptomatic atrial fibrillation: a comparative, placebo controlled study. *Heart.* 2000;84:251–257.

60. Juul-Moller S, Edvardsson N, Rehnqvist-Ahlberg N. Sotalol versus quinidine for the maintenance of sinus rhythm after direct current conversion of atrial fibrillation. *Circulation.* 1990;82:1932–1939.

61. Benditt DG et al., for the d,l-Sotalol Atrial Fibrillation/Flutter Study Group. Maintenance of sinus rhythm with oral d,l-sotalol therapy in patients with symptomatic atrial fibrillation and/or atrial flutter. *Am J Cardiol.* 1999;84:270–277.

62. Wanless RS et al. Multicenter comparative study of the efficacy and safety of sotalol in the prophylactic treatment of patients with paroxysmal supraventricular tachyarrhythmias. *Am Heart J.* 1997;133:441–446.

63. Julian DG et al. Randomized trial of effect of amiodarone on mortality in patients with left-ventricular dysfunction after recent myocardial infarction: EMIAT (European Myocardial Infarct Amiodarone Trial Investigators). *Lancet.* 1997;349:667–674.

64. Cairns JA et al. Randomized trial of outcome after myocardial infarction in patients with frequent or repetitive ventricular premature depolarisations: CAM-IAT. *Lancet.* 1997;349:675–682.

65. Crijins HJ, Gosselink AT, Lie KI, for the PRODIS Study Group. Propafenone versus disopyramide for maintenance of sinus rhythm after electrical cardioversion of chronic atrial fibrillation: a randomized, double-blnd study. *Cardiovasc Drugs Ther.* 1996;10:145–152.

66. Hartel G, Louhija A, Konttinen A. Disopyramide in the prevention of recurrence of atrial fibrillation after electroconversion. *Clin Pharmacol Ther.* 1974;15:551–555.

67. Karlson BW et al. Disopyramide in the maintenance of sinus rhythm after electroconversion of atrial fibrillation: a placebo-controlled one-year follow-up study. *Eur Heart J.* 1988;9:284–290.

68. Lloyd EA, Gersh BJ, Forman R. The efficacy of quinidine and disopyramide in the maintenance of sinus rhythm after electroconversion from atrial fibrillation: a double-blind study comparing quinidine, disopyramide, and placebo. *S Afr Med J.* 1984;65:367–369.

69. Naccarelli GV et al. for the Flecainide Multicenter Atrial Fibrillation Study Group. Prospective comparison of flecainide versus quinidine for the treatment of paroxysmal atrial fibrillation/flutter. *Am J Cardiol.* 1996;77:53A–59A.

70. Van Wijk LM et al. Flecainide versus quinidine in the prevention of paroxysms of atrial fibrillation. *J Cardiovasc Pharmacol.* 1989;13:32–36.

71. Pietersen AH, Hellemann H, for the Danish-Norwegian Flecainide Multicenter Study Group. Usefulness of flecainide for prevention of paroxysmal atrial fibrillation and flutter. *Am J Cardiol.* 1991;67:713–717.

72. Clementry J et al. Flecainide acetate in the prevention of paroxysmal atrial fibrillation: a nine-month follow-up of more than 500 patients. *Am J Cardiol.* 1992;70:44A–49A.

73. Sonnhag C et al. Long-term efficacy of flecainide in paroxysmal atrial fibrillation. *Acta Med Scand.* 1988;224:563–569.

74. Van Gelder IC et al. Efficacy and safety of flecainide acetate in the maintenance of sinus rhythm after electrical conversion of chronic atrial fibrillation or atrial flutter. *Am J Cardiol.* 1989;64:1317–1321.

75. UK Propafenone PSVT Study Group. A randomized, placebo-controlled trial of propafenone in the prophylaxis of paroxysmal supraventricular tachycardia and paroxysmal atrial fibrillation. *Circulation.* 1995;92:2550–2557.

76. Connolly SJ, Hoffert DL. Usefulness of propafenone for recurrent paroxysmal atrial fibrillation. *Am J Cardiol.* 1989;63:817–819.

77. Lee SH et al. Comparisons of oral propafenone and quinidine as an initial treatment option in patients with symptomatic paroxysmal atrial fibrillation: a double-blind, randomized trial. *J Intern Med.* 1996;239:253–260.

78. Reimold SC et al. Propafenone versus sotalol for suppression of recurrent symptomatic atrial fibrillation. *Am J Cardiol.* 1993;71:558–563.

79. DiMarco JP et al. Adenosine for paroxysmal supraventricular tachycardia: dose ranging and comparison with verapamil: assessment in placebo-controlled, multicentre trials. *Ann Intern Med.* 1990;113:104–110.

80. DiMarco JP et al. Adenosine: electrophysiologic effects and therapeutic use for terminating paroxysmal suprventricular tachycardia. *Circulation.* 1983;68:1254–1263.

81. Sung RJ, Elser B, McAllister RG. Intravenous verapamil for termination of reentrant supraventricular tachycardia. *Ann Intern Med.* 1980;93:682–689.

82. Dougherty AH et al. Acute conversion of paroxysmal supraventricular tachycardia with intravenous diltiazem: IV Diltiazem Study Group. *Am J Cardiol.* 1992;70:587–592.

83. Moller B, Ringqvist C. Metoprolol in the treatment of supraventricular tachyarrhythmias. *Ann Clin Res.* 1979;11:34–41.

84. Aronow WS. Clinical use of digitalis. *Compr Ther.* 1992;18:38–41.

85. Chapman MJ et al. Management of atrial tachyarrhythmias in the critically ill: a comparison of intravenous procainamide and amiodarone. *Intensive Care Med.* 1993;19:48–52.

86. Vietti-Ramus G et al. Efficacy and safety of short intravenous amiodarone in supraventricular tachyarrhythmias. *Int J Cardiol.* 1992;35:77–85.

87. Holt P et al. Intravenous amiodarone in the acute termination of supraventricular arrhythmias. *Int J Cardiol.* 1985;8:67–79.

88. Cybulski J et al. Intravenous amiodarone is safe and seems to be effective in termination of paroxysmal supraventricular tachyarrhythmias. *Clin Cardiol.* 1996;19:563–566.

89. Jordaens L et al., for the Sotalol Versus Placebo Multicenter Study Group. Efficacy and safety of intravenous sotalol for termination of paroxysmal supraventricular tachycardia. *Am J Cardiol.* 1991;68:35–40.

90. Sung RJ et al., for the Sotalol Multicenter Study Group. Intravenous sotalol for the termination of supraventricular tachycardia and atrial fibrillation and flutter: a multicenter, randomized, double-blind, placebo-controlled study. *Am Heart J.* 1995;129:739–748.

91. Bertini G et al. Propafenone versus amiodarone in field treatment of primary atrial tachydysrhythmias. *J Emerg Med.* 1990;8:15–20.

92. O'Nunain S et al. A comparison of intravenous propafenone and flecainide in the treatment of tachycardias associated with the Wolff-Parkinson-White syndrome. *Pacing Clin Electrophysiol.* 1991;14:2028–2034.

93. Levine J, Michael J, Guarnieri T. Treatment of multifocal atrial tachycardia with verapamil. *New Engl J Med.* 1985;312:21–25.

94. Singh BN, Nademanee K. Use of calcium antagonists for cardiac arrhythmias. *Am J Cardiol.* 1987;59:153B–62B.

95. Arsura E et al. A randomized, double-blind, placebo-controlled study of verapamil and metoprolol in treatment of multifocal atrial tachycardia. *Am J Med.* 1988;85:519–524.

96. Kouvaras G et al. The effective treatment of multifocal atrial tachycardia with amiodarone. *Jpn Heart J.* 1989;30:301–312.

97. Latini R, Maggioni AP, Cavalli A. Therapeutic drug monitoring of antiarrhythmic drugs: rationale and current status. *Clin Pharmacokinet.* 1990;18:91–103.

98. Podrid PJ, Schoeneberger A, Lown B. Congestive heart failure caused by oral disopyramide. *New Engl J Med.* 1980;302:614–617.

99. Connolly SJ, Kates RE. Clinical pharmacokinetics of N-acetylprocainamide. *Clin Pharmacokinet.* 1982;7:206–220.

100. Karlsson E. Clinical pharmacokinetics of procainamide. *Clin Pharmacokinet.* 1978;3:97–107.

101. Strasberg B et al. Procainamide-induced polymorphous ventricular tachyardia. *Am J Cardiol.* 1981;47:1309–1314.

102. Greenblatt DJ, Pfeifer HJ, Ochs HR, et al. Pharmacokinetics of quinidine in humans after intravenous, intramuscular and oral administration. *J Pharmacol Exp Ther.* 1977;202:365–378.

103. Oberg KC et al. "Late" proarrhythmia due to quinidine. *Am J Cardiol.* 1994;74:192–194.

104. Gross AS et al. Polymorphic flecainide disposition under conditions of uncontrolled urine flow and pH. *Eur J Clin Pharmacol.* 1991;40:155–162.

105. Conrad GJ, Ober RE. Metabolism of flecainide. *Am J Cardiol.* 1984;53:41B–51B.

106. Holmes B, Heel RC. Flecianide: a preliminary review of its pharmacodynamic properties and therapeutic efficacy. *Drugs.* 1985;29:1–33.

107. Echt DS et al. Mortality and morbidity in patients receiving encainide, flecainide, or placebo. The Cardiac Arrhythmia Suppression Trial. *New Engl J Med.* 1991;324:781–788.

108. Siddoway LA et al. Polymorphism of propafenone metabolism and disposition in man: clinical and pharmacokinetic consequences. *Circulation.* 1987;75: 785–791.

109. Parker RB, McCollam PL, Bauman JL. Propafenone: a novel type Ic antiarrhythmic agent. *DICP.* 1989;23:196–202.

110. Angaran DM, Schultz NJ, Tschida VH. Esmolol hydrochloride: an ultrashort-acting β-adrenergic blocking agent. *Clin Pharmacol.* 1986;5:288–303.

111. Roden DM. Pharmacokinetics of amiodarone: implications for drug therapy. *Am J Cardiol.* 1993;72:45F–50F.

112. Gill J, Heel RC, Fitton A. Amiodarone: an overview of its pharmacologic properties, and review of its therapeutic use in cardiac arrhythmias. *Drugs.* 1992;43:69–110.

113. Rotmensch HH, Rocci ML, Vlasses PH. Steady-state serum amiodarone concentrations: relationship with antiarrhythmic efficacy and toxicity. *Ann Intern Med.* 1984;101:462–469.

114. Desai AD, Chun S, Sung RJ. The role of intravenous amiodarone in the management of cardiac arrhythmias. *Ann Intern Med.* 1997;127:294–303.

115. Goldschlager N et al. Practical guidelines for clinicians who treat patients with amiodarone. *Arch Intern Med.* 2000;160:1741–1748.

116. Lenz TL, Hilleman DE. Dofetilide: a new class III antiarrhythmic agent. *Pharmacotherapy,* 2000;20:776-86.

117. Kalus JS, Mauro VF. Dofetilide: a class III-specific antiarrhythmic agent. *Ann Pharmacother.* 2000;34:44–56.

118. Howard PA. Ibutilide: an antiarrhythmic agent for the treatment of atrial fibrillation or flutter. *Ann Pharmacother.* 1999;33:38–47.

119. Kowey PR, VanderLugt JT, Luderer JR. Safety and risk/benefit analysis of ibutilide for acute conversion of atrial fibrillation/flutter. *Am J Cardiol.* 1996;78(suppl 8A):46–52.

120. Hanyok JJ. Clinical pharmacokinetics of sotalol. *Am J Cardiol.* 1993;72:19A–26A.

121. MacNeil DJ, Davies RO, Deitchman D. Clinical safety profile of sotalol in the treatment of arrhythmias. *Am J Cardiol.* 1993;72:44A–50A.

122. Smith MS et al. Pharmacokinetic and pharmacodynamic effects of diltiazem. *Am J Cardiol.* 1983;51:1369–1374.

123. Barbarash RA et al. Verapamil infusions in the treatment of atrial tachyarrhythmias. *Crit Care Med.* 1986;14:886–888.

124. Hamann SR, Blouin RA, McAllister RG. Clinical pharmacokinetics of verapamil. *Clin Pharmacokinet.* 1984;9:26–41.

125. McIntosh-Yellin NL, Drew BJ, Scheinman MM. Safety and efficacy of central intravenous bolus administration of adenosine for termination of supraventricular tachycardia. *J Am Coll Cardiol.* 1993;22:741–745.

126. Lisalo E. Clinical pharmacokinetics of digoxin. *Clin Pharmacokinet.* 1977;2:1–16.

127. Jelliffe RW. An improved method of digoxin therapy. *Ann Intern Med.* 1968;69:703–717.

128. Ewy GA et al. Digitalis intoxication: diagnosis, management, and prevention. *Cardiol Clin.* 1974;6:153–174.

129. Kerin NZ et al. The incidence, magnitude, and time course of the amiodarone-Warfarin interaction. *Arch Intern Med.* 1998;148:1779–1781.

130. O'Reilly RA et al. Interaction of amiodarone with racemic Warfarin and its separated enantiomorphs in humans. *Clin Pharmacol Ther.* 1987;42:290–294.

131. Watt AH et al. Amiodarone reduces plasma Warfarin clearance in man. *Br J Clin Pharmac.* 1985;20:707–709.

132. Hamer A et al. The potentiation of Warfarin anticoagulation by amiodarone. *Circulation.* 1982;65:1025–1029.

133. Cheung B, Lam FM, Kumana CR. Insidiously evolving, occult drug interaction involving Warfarin and amiodarone. *Br Med J.* 1996;312:107–108.

134. Sanoski CA, Bauman JL. Clinical observations with the amiodarone/Warfarin interaction: dosing relationships with long-term therapy. *Chest.* 2002;121:19–23.

135. Nademanee K et al. Amiodarone-digoxin interaction: clinical significance, time course of development, potential pharmacokinetic mechanisms and therapeutic implications. *J Am Coll Cardiol.* 1984;4:111–116.

136. Chitwood KK, Abdul-Hagg AJ, Heim-Duthoy KL. Cyclosporine-amiodarone interaction. *Ann Pharmacother.* 1993;27:569–571.

137. Nolan PE et al. Steady-state interaction betweeen amiodarone and phenytoin. *Am J Cardiol.* 1990;65:1252–1257.

138. Liu LL, Knowlton PW, Svensson CK. Effect of amiodarone on the disposition of procainamide in the rat. *J Pharm Sci*. 1988;77:662–665.

139. Tartini R et al. Dangerous interaction between amiodarone and quinidine. *Lancet*. 1982;1:1327–1329.

140. Ha HR et al. Interaction between amiodarone and lidocaine. *J Cardiovasc Pharmacol*. 1996;28:533–539.

141. Siegmund JB, Wilson JH, Imhoff TE. Amiodarone interaction with lidocaine. *J Cardiovasc Pharmacol*. 1993;21:513–515.

9 Ventricular Arrhythmias

Cynthia A. Sanoski

CONTENTS

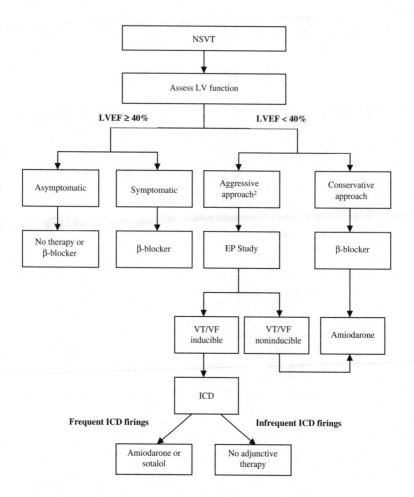

FIGURE 9.1 Algorithm for management of nonsustained ventricular tachycardia. NSVT = non-sustained ventricular tachycardia; LV = left ventricular; LVEF = left ventricular ejection fraction; EP = electrophysiology; VT = ventricular tachycardia; VF = ventricular fibrillation; ICD = implantable cardioverter-defibrillator. (Adapted from Tisdale JE, Moser LR, In: Mueller BA et al., eds. *Pharmacotherapy Self-Assessment Program.* 4th ed. Kansas City, MO: ACCP; 2001.)

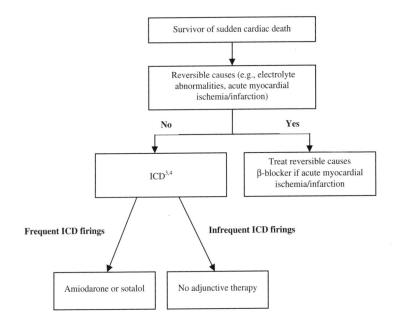

FIGURE 9.2 Algorithm for management of survivors of sudden cardiac death. ICD = implantable cardioverter-defibrillator. (Adapted from Tisdale JE, Moser LR, In: Mueller BA et al., eds. *Pharmacotherapy Self-Assessment Program.* 4th ed. Kansas City, MO: ACCP; 2001.)

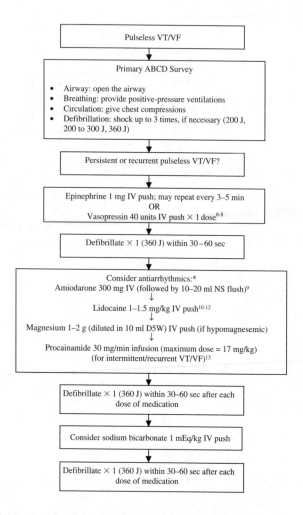

FIGURE 9.3 Algorithm for management of pulseless ventricular tachycardia/ventricular fibrillation. VT = ventricular tachycardia; VF = ventricular fibrillation; J = joules; IV = intravenous; NS = normal saline; D5W = 5% dextrose in water; *See Tables 9.1, 9.2, and 9.4 for additional dosing recommendations. (Adapted from The American Heart Association in Collaboration with the International Liaison Committee on Resuscitation. *Circulation.* 2000;102(Suppl I):I-142.)

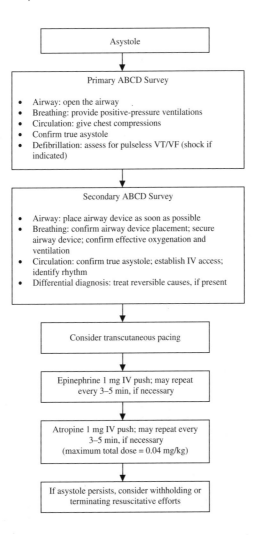

FIGURE 9.4 Algorithm for management of asystole. VT = ventricular tachycardia; VF = ventricular fibrillation; IV = intravenous. (Adapted from The American Heart Association in Collaboration with the International Liaison Committee on Resuscitation. *Circulation.* 2000;102(Suppl I):I-142.)

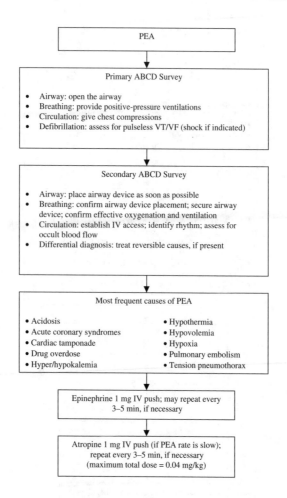

FIGURE 9.5 Algorithm for management of pulseless electrical activity. PEA = pulseless electrical activity; VT = ventricular tachycardia; VF = ventricular fibrillation; IV = intravenous. (Adapted from The American Heart Association in Collaboration with the International Liaison Committee on Resuscitation. *Circulation.* 2000;102(Suppl I):I-142.)

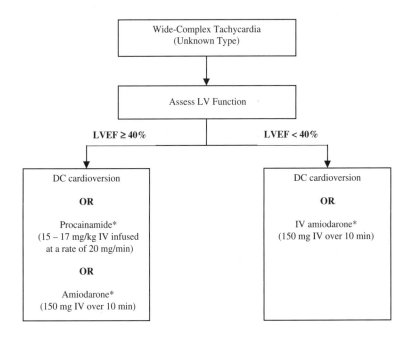

FIGURE 9.6 Algorithm for hemodynamically stable wide-complex tachycardia (unknown type). LV = left ventricular; LVEF = left ventricular ejection fraction; DC = direct current; IV = intravenous; *See Tables 9.1 and 9.4 for additional dosing recommendations. (Adapted from The American Heart Association in Collaboration with the International Liaison Committee on Resuscitation. *Circulation.* 2000;102(Suppl I):I-158.)

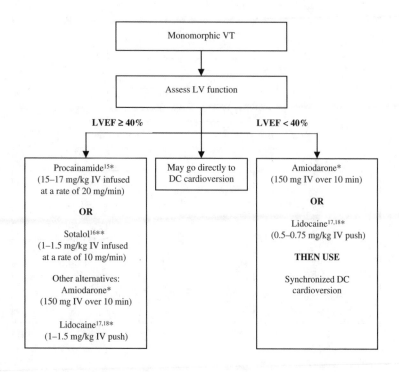

FIGURE 9.7 Algorithm for hemodynamically stable monomorphic ventricular tachycardia. VT = ventricular tachycardia; LV = left ventricular; LVEF = left ventricular ejection fraction; IV = intravenous; DC = direct current; *See Tables 9.1, 9.2, and 9.4 for additional dosing recommendations; **IV sotalol is not available in the United States. (Adapted from The American Heart Association in Collaboration with the International Liaison Committee on Resuscitation. *Circulation.* 2000;102(Suppl I):I-158.)

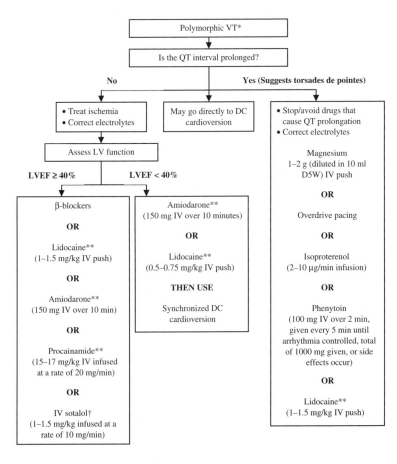

FIGURE 9.8 Algorithm for hemodynamically stable polymorphic ventricular tachycardia. *Hemodynamically unstable polymorphic ventricular tachycardia should be treated using the pulseless ventricular tachycardia/ventricular fibrillation algorithm; **See Tables 9.1, 9.2, and 9.4 for additional dosing recommendations; † IV sotalol is not available in the United States; VT = ventricular tachycardia; DC = direct current; LV = left ventricular; LVEF = left ventricular ejection fraction; IV = intravenous; D5W = 5% dextrose in water. (Adapted from The American Heart Association in Collaboration with the International Liaison Committee on Resuscitation. *Circulation.* 2000;102(Suppl I):I-158.)

TABLE 9.1
Class Ia Antiarrhythmics

Drug	Half-Life	Route of Elimination	Usual Dose	Maximum Dose	Therapeutic Range	Adverse Effects	Monitoring Parameters	Ref.
Disopyramide	4–10 h	Hepatic/renal	<50 kg: IR: 100 mg po q 6 h CR: 200 mg po q 12 h >50 kg: IR: 150 mg po q 6 h CR: 300 mg po 12 h Renal insufficiency (only use IR form): CrCl 30–40 ml/min: 100 mg po q 8 h CrCl 15–30 ml/min: 100 mg po q 12 h CrCl < 15 ml/min: 100 mg po q 24 h	<50 kg: 400 mg/day >50 kg: 400 mg po q 6 h (IR)	2–5 µg/ml	Nausea, anorexia, dry mouth, urinary retention, blurred vision, constipation, heart failure exacerbation, torsades de pointes, hypotension	ECG (QTc interval, QRS duration), BP, signs/symptoms of heart failure, electrolytes (K$^+$, Mg^{2+})	19, 20

| Procainamide | PA: 2.5–5 h[a] NAPA: 6–8 h | Hepatic/renal PA: ~15–30% eliminated renally as unchanged drug; remainder metabolized in liver to NAPA NAPA: Renally eliminated | IV: Refractory VT/VF: 15–17 mg/kg infused at 30 mg/min (max total dose = 17 mg/kg) Stable VT: 20 mg/min infusion given until arrhythmia suppressed, hypotension occurs, QRS widens by >50%, or total dose of 17 mg/kg is given MD = 1–4 mg/min continuous infusion PO: Usual dose: 50 mg/kg/day IR: 250–500 mg po q 3–6 h Procan SR®: 500–1000 mg po q 6 h Procanbid®. 500–2000 mg q 12 h | Should be adjusted for each patient individually based upon renal function, plasma levels, and therapeutic response. Use with caution, if at all, in renal insufficiency | PA: 4–10 μg/ml NAPA: 15–25 μg/ml Total: 10–30 μg/ml | Diarrhea, nausea, vomiting, SLE-like syndrome (rash, arthralgias, fever, pericarditis, pleuritis), torsades de pointes, hypotension (with IV), agranulocytosis | ECG (QTc interval, QRS duration), BP, PA/NAPA levels, CBC with differential, electrolytes (K^+, Mg^{2+}) | 5, 21–23 |

TABLE 9.1 (CONTINUED)
Class Ia Antiarrhythmics

Drug	Half-Life	Route of Elimination	Usual Dose	Maximum Dose	Therapeutic Range	Adverse Effects	Monitoring Parameters	Ref.
Quinidine	6–8 h	Hepatic	Quinidine sulfate: 200–400 mg po q 6 h Quinidine gluconate: 324 mg po q 8–12 h	Quinidine sulfate: 600 mg po q 6 h Quinidine gluconate: 972 mg po q 8–12 h	2–5 µg/ml	Torsades de pointes, diarrhea, stomach cramps, nausea, vomiting, hypotension, fever, thrombocytopenia, cinchonism (tinnitus, blurred vision, headache)	ECG (QTc interval, QRS duration), BP, quinidine levels, CBC, liver function tests, electrolytes (K^+, Mg^{2+})	24, 25

IR = immediate release; CR = controlled release; CrCl = creatinine clearance; ECG = electrocardiogram; QTc interval = corrected QT interval; BP = blood pressure; K^+ = potassium; Mg^{2+} = magnesium; PA = procainamide; NAPA = N-acetyl procainamide; IV = intravenous; VT = ventricular tachycardia; VF = ventricular fibrillation; MD = maintenance dose; po = oral; SR = sustained release; SLE = systemic lupus erythematosus; CBC = complete blood count.

[a] PA half-life also depends on acetylator phenotype (fast vs. slow).

TABLE 9.2
Class Ib Antiarrhythmics

Drug	Half-Life	Route of Elimination	Usual Dose	Maximum Dose	Therapeutic Range	Adverse Effects	Monitoring Parameters	Ref.
Lidocaine	1.5–2 h	Hepatic	Pulseless VT/VF: 1–1.5 mg/kg IV push; may give additional 0.5–0.75 mg/kg IV push in 3–5 min, if necessary (maximum total dose = 3 mg/kg) Stable VT: LVEF > 40%: Same as above for pulseless VT/VF LVEF < 40%: 0.5–0.75 mg/kg IV push; may repeat every 5–10 min, if necessary (maximum total dose =3 mg/kg) MD = 1–2 mg/min continuous infusion	Maximum total LD: 3 mg/kg; lower initial MD should be used in patients with heart failure or hepatic disease	1.5–5 μg/ml	Dizziness, nausea, vomiting, drowsiness, slurred speech, blurred vision, paresthesias, muscle twitching, confusion, hallucinations, psychosis, vertigo, tinnitus, seizures, bradycardia, respiratory depression	ECG (QRS duration), lidocaine levels, BP, HR, RR; especially monitor levels and signs/ symptoms of toxicity in patients with heart failure, hepatic disease, acute MI, or in those receiving therapy for >24 h	5, 26, 27

TABLE 9.2 (CONTINUED)
Class Ib Antiarrhythmics

Drug	Half-Life	Route of Elimination	Usual Dose	Maximum Dose	Therapeutic Range	Adverse Effects	Monitoring Parameters	Ref.
Mexiletine	10–14 h	Hepatic	Initial: 200 mg po q 8 h; may adjust dose every 2–3 days Usual dose = 200–300 mg po q 8 h Maintenance dose should be reduced by 30–50% in patients with heart failure or hepatic disease; should be administered with food to minimize gastrointestinal symptoms	400 mg po q 8 h	Not monitored clinically	Lightheadedness, dizziness, drowsiness, nervousness, confusion, paresthesias, tremor, ataxia, weakness, blurred vision, nystagmus, tinnitus, nausea, vomiting, anorexia, ventricular arrhythmias, seizures	ECG (QRS duration), BP, HR, liver function tests; especially monitor signs/symptoms of toxicity in patients with heart failure or hepatic disease	28, 29

VT = ventricular tachycardia; VF = ventricular fibrillation; IV = intravenous; LVEF = left ventricular ejection fraction; MD = maintenance dose; LD = loading dose; ECG = electrocardiogram; BP = blood pressure; HR = heart rate; RR = respiratory rate; MI = myocardial infarction.

TABLE 9.3
Class Ic Antiarrhythmics

Drug	Half-Life	Primary Route of Elimination	Usual Dose	Maximum Dose	Therapeutic Range	Adverse Effects	Monitoring Parameters	Ref.
Flecainide	7–22 h	Hepatic/renal	Initial dose: 100 mg po q 12 h; increase by 50–100 mg/day every 4 days until desired response Patients with renal insufficiency: CrCl <35 ml/min: Reduce initial dose to 50 mg po q 12 h	200 mg po every 12 h	Not monitored clinically	Dizziness, visual disturbances, dyspnea, headache, tremor, nausea, heart failure exacerbation, ventricular tachycardia	ECG (QRS duration), baseline echocardiogram (to evaluate left ventricular function)	30–33
Propafenone	Extensive metabolizers (90% of patients): 2–8 h Poor metabolizers (10% of patients): 10–32 h	Hepatic	150 mg po every 8 h	300 mg po every 8 h	Not monitored clinically	Bradycardia, AV block, heart failure exacerbation, ventricular tachycardia, nausea, vomiting, dizziness, fatigue, bronchospasm, headache, taste disturbances	ECG (QRS duration, PR interval), HR, BP, baseline echocardiogram (to evaluate left ventricular function)	34, 35

CrCl = creatinine clearance; ECG = electrocardiogram; HR = heart rate; BP = blood pressure.

TABLE 9.4
Class III Antiarrhythmics

Drug	Half-Life	Primary Route of Elimination	Usual Dose	Maximum Dose	Therapeutic Range	Adverse Effects	Monitoring Parameters	Ref.
Amiodarone	40–55 days (range = 25–107 days)	Hepatic	IV: See Table 9.5 PO: See Table 9.5	LD should be given until patient has received ~15 g; the dose can then be tapered to the MD regimen	1–2 mg/l (serum levels have not been shown to correlate with clinical efficacy)	IV: Hypotension, bradycardia, heart block, phlebitis PO: Hypothyroidism, hyperthyroidism, pulmonary fibrosis, bradycardia, heart block, corneal microdeposits, optic neuritis, nausea, vomiting, anorexia, constipation, ↑ LFTs, hepatitis, tremor, ataxia, paresthesias, photosensitivity, blue-gray skin discoloration, insomnia	ECG (QTc interval, QRS duration, PR interval), HR, BP, CXR, PFTs, TFTs, LFTs, ophthalmologic exam (see Table 8.8 for monitoring guidelines)	5, 35–39

| Sotalol | 12 h | Renal | Initial: 80 mg po bid; dose can be increased at 2–3 day intervals to maximum of 320 mg po bid Dosing interval must be adjusted in patients with renal insufficiency: CrCl 30–60 ml/min: every 24 h CrCl 10–29 ml/min:every 36–48 h CrCl < 10 ml/min: contraindicated | 320 mg po bid Higher doses (480–640 mg/day) should be reserved for patients with drug-refractory ventricular arrhythmias | Not monitored clinically | Torsades de pointes, bradycardia, chest pain, palpitations, fatigue, light-headedness, weakness, dyspnea, bronchospasm, heart failure exacerbation, nausea, vomiting, diarrhea | ECG (QTc interval, PR interval), HR, electrolytes (K^+, Mg^{2+}), | 41, 42 |

IV = intravenous; po = oral; LD = loading dose; MD = maintenance dose; LFTs = liver function tests; ECG = electrocardiogram; QTc interval = corrected QT interval; HR = heart rate; BP = blood pressure; CXR = chest x-ray; PFTs = pulmonary function tests; TFTs = thyroid function tests; bid = twice daily; CrCl = creatinine clearance; K^+ = potassium; Mg^{2+} = magnesium.

TABLE 9.5
Amiodarone Dosing for Ventricular Arrhythmias

Intravenous Amiodarone

Pulseless VT/VF:

Loading dose	300 mg IV push (followed by 10–20 ml NS flush); may repeat with 150 mg IV push every 3–5 min, if necessary (followed by 10–20 ml NS flush)
Maintenance dose (if stable rhythm achieved)	1 mg/min continuous infusion for 6 h, then 0.5 mg/min; maximum dose = 2.2 g/24 h; convert patient to oral therapy when hemodynamically stable and able to take oral medications

Stable VT:

Loading dose	150 mg IV (diluted in 100 ml D5W or NS) over 10 min; may repeat dose every 10 min, if necessary, for breakthrough VT
Maintenance dose	1 mg/min continuous infusion for 6 h, then 0.5 mg/min; maximum dose = 2.2 g/24 h; convert patient to oral therapy when hemodynamically stable and able to take oral medications

Oral Amiodarone

Loading dose	1200–1600 mg/day in 2–3 divided doses for 1 week (until patient receives ~15 g total load), then give MD Loading doses should be administered with food to minimize gastrointestinal symptoms
Maintenance dose	300–400 mg po qd; patients with an ICD who require adjunctive antiarrhythmic therapy may only require an MD of 200 mg/day to further suppress ventricular arrhythmias

TABLE 9.5 (CONTINUED)
Amiodarone Dosing for Ventricular Arrhythmias

Guidelines for Converting from IV to Oral Therapy

Duration of IV Amiodarone Infusion	Initial Daily Dose of Oral Amiodarone
<1 week	1200–1600 mg[a]
1–3 weeks	600–800 mg[a]
>3 weeks	400 mg

VT = ventricular tachycardia; VF = ventricular fibrillation; IV = intravenous; NS = normal saline; D5W = 5% dextrose in water; MD = maintenance dose; qd = every day; ICD = implantable cardioverter-defibrillator.

[a] These daily doses should be continued until patient has received ~15 g total load. Paient can then be given MD.

TABLE 9.6
Follow-Up Plans for Ventricular Arrhythmias

Acute Therapy

Heart rate, blood pressure, respiratory rate, and rhythm should be closely monitored.

- Patient should be on telemetry throughout the hospitalization to monitor for recurrence of the arrhythmia.
- Measure QRS duration, QTc interval, and PR interval.

Monitor for adverse effects associated with intravenous amiodarone, lidocaine, and procainamide.

Lidocaine levels should be monitored under the following circumstances:

- Patient has condition that alters the disposition of lidocaine (e.g., heart failure, hepatic dysfunction, acute myocardial infarction).
- Toxicity is suspected.
- Prolonged therapy (>24 h) is required.
- Concomitant therapy with an interacting drug (e.g., amiodarone).

Procainamide levels should be monitored under the following circumstances:

- Patient has condition that alters the disposition of procainamide (e.g., renal or hepatic dysfunction).
- Toxicity is suspected.
- Prolonged therapy (>24 h) is required.
- Concomitant therapy with an interacting drug (e.g., amiodarone).

Plasma amiodarone and/or desethylamiodarone concentrations do not need to be monitored as there does not appear to be a relationship between these concentrations and the clinical efficacy of the drug.

Chronic Therapy

Heart rate, blood pressure, and rhythm should be routinely monitored in patients receiving long-term antiarrhythmic therapy.

- Measure QRS duration, QTc interval, and PR interval.

Patients receiving sotalol should have their renal function monitored on a regular basis. If the patient devlops renal dysfunction (CrCl <60 ml/min), either the dose of sotalol should be adjusted or another antiarrhythmic should be used.

Patients receiving amiodarone should be routinely monitored for amiodarone-induced adverse effects and drug interactions.

- See Table 8.8 for monitoring guidelines.
- Educate patient on signs/symptoms of adverse effects associated with amiodarone.

TABLE 9.6 (CONTINUED)
Follow-Up Plans for Ventricular Arrhythmias

Chronic Therapy (Continued)

Plasma amiodarone and/or desethylamiodarone concentrations do not need to be monitored as there does not appear to be a relationship between these concentrations and the clinical efficacy of the drug.

The efficacy of any adjunctive antiarrhythmic therapy should be routinely monitored in patients with an implantable cardioverter-defibrillator by evaluating the number of shocks that the patient receives.

Patients should be educated on the importance of medication compliance.

REFERENCES

1. Tisdale JE, Moser LR. Tachyarrhythmias. In: Mueller BA, Bertch KE, Dunswort TS, eds. *Pharmacotherapy Self-Assessment Program*, 4th ed. Kansas City, MO: ACCP; 2001.

2. Buxton AE et al. A randomized study of the prevention of sudden death in patients with coronary artery disease. *New Engl J Med.* 1999;341:1882–1890.

3. The Antiarrhythmics Versus Implantable Defibrillators (AVID) Investigators. A comparison of antiarrhythmic-drug therapy with implantable defibrillators in patients resuscitated from near-fatal ventricular arrhythmias. *New Engl J Med.* 1997;337:1576–1583.

4. Kuck KH et al. Randomized comparison of antiarrhythmic drug therapy with implantable defibrillators in patients resuscitated from cardiac arrest: The Cardiac Arrest Study Hamburg (CASH). *Circulation.* 2000;102:748–754.

5. The American Heart Association in Collaboration with the International Liason Committee on Resuscitation (ILCOR). Guidelines 2000 for Cardiopulmonary Resuscitation and Emergency Cardiovascular Care: An International Consensus on Science. *Circulation.* 2000;102(Suppl I): I-142–I-157.

6. Lindner KH et al. Vasopressin administration in refractory cardiac arrest. *Ann Intern Med.* 1996;124:1061–1064.

7. Lindner KH, Dirks B, Strohmenger HU. Randomized comparison of epinephrine and vasopressin in patients with out-of-hospital ventricular fibrillation. *Lancet.* 1997;349:535–537.

8. Stiell IG et al. Vasopressin versus epinephrine for inhospital cardiac arrest: a randomised controlled trial. *Lancet.* 2001;358:105–109.

9. Kudenchuck PJ et al. Amiodarone for resuscitation after out-of-hospital cardiac arrest due to ventricular fibrillation. *New Engl J Med.* 1999;341:871–879.

10. Harrison EE. Lidocaine in prehospital coutershock refractory ventricular fibrillation. *Ann Emerg Med.* 1981;10:420–423.

11. Haynes RE et al. Comparison of bretylium tosylate and lidocaine in management of out of hospital ventricular fibrillation: a randomized clinical trial. *Am J Cardiol.* 1981;48:353–356.

12. Olson DW et al. A randomized comparison study of bretylium tosylate and lidocaine in resuscitation of patients from out-of-hospital ventricular fibrillation in a paramedic system. *Ann Emerg Med.* 1984;13:807–810.

13. Stiell IG et al. Association of drug therapy with survival in cardiac arrest: limited role of advanced cardiac life support drugs. *Acad Emerg Med.* 1995;2:264–273.

14. The American Heart Association in Collaboration with the International Liaison Committee on Resuscitation (ILCOR). Guidelines 2000 for Cardiopulmonary Resuscitation and Emergency Cardiovascular Care: An International Consensus on Science. *Circulation.* 2000;102(Suppl I): I-158–I-165.

15. Gorgels AP et al. Comparison of procainamide and lidocaine in terminating sustained monomorphic ventricular tachycardia. *Am J Cardiol.* 1996;78:43–46.

16. Ho DS et al. Double-blind trial of lignocaine versus sotalol for acute termination of spontaneous sustained ventricular tachycardia. *Lancet.* 1994;344:18–23.

17. Armengol RE et al. Lack of effectiveness of lidocaine for sustained, wide QRS complex tachycardia. *Ann Emerg Med.* 1989;18:254–257.

18. Nasir N et al. Evaluation of intravenous lidocaine for the termination of sustained monomorphic ventricular tachycardia in patients with coronary artery disease with or without healed myocardial infarction. *Am J Cardiol.* 1994;74:1183–1186.

19. Latini R, Maggioni AP, Cavalli A. Therapeutic drug monitoring of antiarrhythmic drugs: rationale and current status. *Clin Pharmacokinet.* 1990;18:91–103.

20. Podrid PJ, Schoeneberger A, Lown B. Congestive heart failure caused by oral disopyramide. *New Engl J Med.* 1980;302:614–617.

21. Connolly SJ, Kates RE. Clinical pharmacokinetics of *N*-acetylprocainamide. *Clin Pharmacokinet.* 1982;7:206–220.

22. Karlsson E. Clinical pharmacokinetics of procainamide. *Clin Pharmacokinet.* 1978;3:97–107.

23. Strasberg B et al. Procainamide-induced polymorphous ventricular tachyardia. *Am J Cardiol.* 1981;47:1309–1314.

24. Greenblatt DJ et al. Pharmacokinetics of quinidine in humans after intravenous, intramuscular and oral administration. *J Pharmacol Exp Ther.* 1977;202: 365–378.

25. Oberg KC et al. "Late" proarrhythmia due to quinidine. *Am J Cardiol.* 1994;74:192–194.

26. Benowitz NL, Meister W. Clinical pharmacokinetics of lignocaine. *Clin Pharmacokinet.* 1978;3:177–201.

27. Thomson PD et al. Lidocaine pharmacokinetics in advanced heart failure, liver disease, and renal failure in humans. *Ann Intern Med.* 1973;78:499–508.

28. Schrader BJ, Bauman JL. Mexiletine: a new type I antiarrhythmic agent. *Drug Intell Clin Pharm.* 1986;20:255–260.

29. Campbell NP et al. The clinical pharmacology of mexiletine. *Br J Clin Pharmacol.* 1978;6:103–108.
30. Gross AS et al. Polymorphic flecianide disposition under conditions of uncontrolled urine flow and pH. *Eur J Clin Pharmacol.* 1991;40:155–162.
31. Conrad GJ, Ober RE. Metabolism of flecainide. *Am J Cardiol.* 1984;53: 41B–51B.
32. Holmes B, Heel RC. Flecianide: a preliminary review of its pharmacodynamic properties and therapeutic efficacy. *Drugs.* 1985;29:1–33.
33. Echt DS, Liebson PR, Mitcvhell LB, et al. Mortality and morbidity in patients receiving encainide, flecainide, or placebo. The Cardiac Arrhythmia Suppression Trial. *New Engl J Med.* 1991;324:781–788.
34. Siddoway LA et al. Polymorphism of propafenone metabolism and disposition in man: clinical and pharmacokinetic consequences. *Circulation.* 1987;75: 785–791.
35. Parker RB, McCollam PL, Bauman JL. Propafenone: a novel type Ic antiarrhythmic agent. *DICP.* 1989;23:196–202.
36. Roden DM. Pharmacokinetics of amiodarone: implications for drug therapy. *Am J Cardiol.* 1993;72:45F–50F.
37. Podrid PJ. Amiodarone: reevaluation of an old drug. *Ann Intern Med.* 1995;122:689–700.
38. Rotmensch HH, Rocci ML, Vlasses PH. Steady-state serum amiodarone concentrations: relationship with antiarrhythmic efficacy and toxicity. *Ann Intern Med.* 1984;101:462–469.
39. Desai AD, Chun S, Sung RJ. The role of intravenous amiodarone in the management of cardiac arrhythmias. *Ann Intern Med.* 1997;127:294–303.
40. Goldschlager N et al. Practical guidelines for clinicians who treat patients with amiodarone. *Arch Intern Med.* 2000;160:1741–1748.
41. Hanyok JJ. Clinical pharmacokinetics of sotalol. *Am J Cardiol.* 1993;72: 19A–26A.
42. MacNeil DJ, Davies RO, Deitchman D. Clinical safety profile of sotalol in the treatment of arrhythmias. *Am J Cardiol.* 1993;72:44A–50A.

10 Pharmacological Management of Thromboembolic Diseases

James Nawarskas

CONTENTS

0-58716-044-7/03/$0.00+$1.50
© 2003 by CRC Press LLC

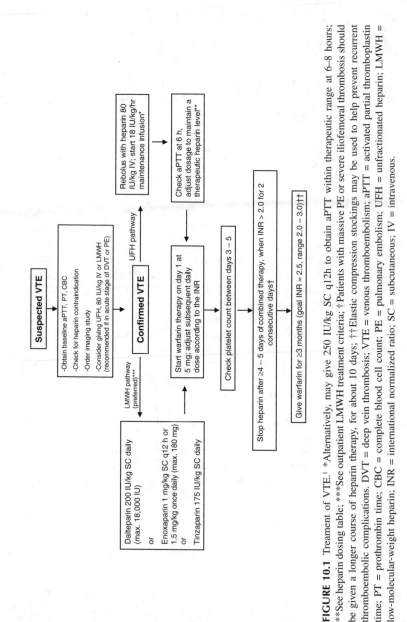

FIGURE 10.1 Treatment of VTE.[1] *Alternatively, may give 250 IU/kg SC q12h to obtain aPTT within therapeutic range at 6–8 hours; **See heparin dosing table; ***See outpatient LMWH treatment criteria; †Patients with massive PE or severe iliofemoral thrombosis should be given a longer course of heparin therapy, for about 10 days; ††Elastic compression stockings may be used to help prevent recurrent thromboembolic complications. DVT = deep vein thrombosis; VTE = venous thromboembolism; aPTT = activated partial thromboplastin time; PT = prothrombin time; CBC = complete blood cell count; PE = pulmonary embolism; UFH = unfractionated heparin; LMWH = low-molecular-weight heparin; INR = international normalized ratio; SC = subcutaneous; IV = intravenous.

Criteria for Outpatient Venous Thromboembolism Treatment with Low-Molecular-Weight Heparin[1]

- Stable proximal deep vein thrombosis or pulmonary embolism
- Normal vital signs
- Low bleeding risk
- Absence of severe renal insufficiency
- Availability of a practical system for administering low-molecular-weight heparin and Warfarin, with appropriate monitoring

---

TABLE 10.1
Weight-Based Dosing of IV Heparin[a]

aPTT (s)	Dose Change (IU/kg/h)	Additional Action	Next aPTT (h)
<35 (1.2 × control)	+4	Rebolus with 80 IU/kg	6
35–45 (1.2–1.5 × control)	+2	Rebolus with 40 IU/kg	6
46–70 (1.5–2.3 × control)	0	—	6; repeat q6h × 24 h then QAM unless outside therapeutic range
71–90 (2.3–3.0 × control)	–2	—	6
>90 (>3 × control)	–3	Stop infusion for 1 h	6

[a] Based on initial dosage of 80 IU/kg bolus followed by 18 IU/kg/h, with aPTT in 6 h.

IV = intravenous; aPTT = activated partial thromboplastin time.

Source: Sixth ACCP Consensus Conference on Antithrombic Therapy: Quick Reference Guide for Clinicians. American College of Chest Physicians; 2001. With permission.

TABLE 10.2
Long-Term Treatment of VTE[1]

Patient Characteristics	Treatment
Most patients	Warfarin for ≥3 months (INR 2–3); use UFH or LMWH for patients unable to take Warfarin
First event, with a reversible or time-limited risk factor (e.g., surgery, trauma, immobilization, estrogen use)	Warfarin ≥3 months*
First episode of idiopathic VTE	Warfarin ≥6 months*
Recurrent idiopathic VTE, or a continuing risk factor (e.g., cancer, antithrombin deficiency, anticardiolipin antibody syndrome)	Warfarin ≥12 months*
Symptomatic isolated calf thrombosis	Warfarin for ≥6 to 12 weeks*; perform serial noninvasive studies of the lower extremity to assess for thrombus extension in patients unable to take anticoagulants
Proximal vein thrombosis or PE or with high risk for these conditions, when anticoagulant therapy is contraindicated or has resulted in a complication	IVC filter
Recurrent thromboembolism despite adequate anticoagulation, chronic recurrent embolism and pulmonary hypertension, and concurrent surgical pulmonary embolectomy or pulmonary thromboendarterectomy	IVC filter

* May use UFH or LMWH if Warfarin cannot be given.

VTE = venous thromboembolism; UFH = unfractionated heparin; LMWH = low-molecular-weight heparin; IVC = inferior vena caval.

Source: *Sixth ACCP Consensus Conference on Antithrombic Therapy: Quick Reference Guide for Clinicians.* American College of Chest Physicians; 2001. With permission.

TABLE 10.3
Antithrombotic Therapy for Valvular Heart Disease[2]

Condition	Recommendation
Mitral Stenosis/Mitral Regurgitation	
History of systemic embolism or presence of atrial fibrillation	Long-term Warfarin (INR 2–3)
NSR, left atrial diameter >5.5 cm	Consider long-term Warfarin (INR 2–3) based on risk factors for thromboembolism, especially left atrial size, patient's age, and hemodynamic severity of the lesion
Recurrent systemic embolism, despite adequate Warfarin therapy	Increase goal INR to 3.0 (range 2.5–3.5), or add aspirin (80–100 mg/day); add dipyridamole (400 mg/day), ticlopidine (250 mg bid), or clopidogrel (75 mg/day) for patient intolerant of aspirin
Mitral Valve Prolapse	
No systemic embolism, unexplained TIA, or atrial fibrillation	**No** anticoagulation
Documented, unexplained TIA	Long-term aspirin (160–325 mg daily)
Documented systemic embolism or recurrent TIA, despite aspirin therapy	Long-term Warfarin (INR 2–3)
Atrial fibrillation despite aspirin therapy	Long-term Warfarin (INR 2–3)
Aortic Valve and Aortic Arch Disorders	
Mobile aortic atheroma and aortic plaque >4 mm, measured by TEE	Long-term Warfarin (INR 2–3)
No other indication for anticoagulation	**No** anticoagulation
Patent Foramen Ovale and Atrial Septal Aneurysm	
Unexplained systemic embolism or TIA, demonstrable venous thrombosis or PE, and either patent foramen ovale (PFO) or atrial septal aneurysm	Long-term Warfarin, unless venous interruption or PFO closure is considered preferable therapy

TABLE 10.3 (CONTINUED)
Antithrombotic Therapy for Valvular Heart Disease[2]

Condition	Recommendation
Infective Endocarditis	
Mechanical prosthetic valve	Continue long-term Warfarin, unless specific contraindications exist; keep in mind the risk of intracranial hemorrhage is substantial when deciding to pursue anticoagulation
Nonbacterial Thrombotic Endocarditis	
Systemic embolism or PE	Heparin
Disseminated cancer, or debilitating disease, with aseptic vegetations seen on echocardiography	Heparin

INR = international normalized ratio; NSR = normal sinus rhythm; TIA = transient ischemic attack; TEE = transesophageal echocardiogram; PE = pulmonary embolism.

Source: *Sixth ACCP Consensus Conference on Antithrombic Therapy: Quick Reference Guide for Clinicians*. American College of Chest Physicians; 2001. With permission.

TABLE 10.4
Antithrombotic Therapy for Prosthetic Heart Valves[8]

Condition	Recommendation
St. Jude Medical or CarboMedics bileaflet aortic valve; Medtronic-Hall tilting disk aortic valve; left atrium of normal size; NSR	Warfarin (INR 2–3)
Tilting disk valve[a], or bileaflet mechanical valve (examples above) in the mitral position; or bileaflet mechanical valve in the aortic position and atrial fibrillation	Warfarin (INR 2.5–3.5) or Warfarin (INR 2–3) + aspirin 80–100 mg/day
Caged ball or caged disk valve (e.g., Starr-Edwards)	Warfarin (INR 2.5–3.5) + aspirin 80–100 mg/day
Any mechanical valve in the presence of additional risk factors	Warfarin (INR 2.5–3.5) + aspirin 80–100 mg/day
Any mechanical valve in the presence of systemic embolism despite anticoagulant therapy	Warfarin (INR 2.5–3.5) + aspirin 80–100 mg/dat

[a] Examples of tilting disk valves: Medtronic-Hall tilting disk, Björk-Shiley spherical disk, Björk-Shiley Convexo Concave (no longer available), and Sorin Monostrut. There are no investigations with INRs of 2.0–3.0 in Björk-Shiley valves.

INR = international normalized ratio; NSR = normal sinus rhythm.

Source: Sixth ACCP Consensus Conference on Antithrombic Therapy: Quick Reference Guide for Clinicians. American College of Chest Physicians; 2001. With permission.

TABLE 10.5
Antithrombotic Therapy for Bioprosthetic Heart Valves[a8]

Condition	Recommendation
Valve in mitral or aortic position	Warfarin (INR 2–3) for the first 3 months after valve insertion; UFH or LMWH may be used until INR is therapeutic for 2 consecutive days
Atrial fibrillation	Long-term Warfarin (INR 2–3)
Evidence of left atrial thrombus at surgery	Long-term Warfarin (INR 2–3)
Permanent pacemaker	Optional Warfarin (INR 2–3)
History of systemic embolism	Warfarin (INR 2–3) for 3–12 months
Normal sinus rhythm	Long-term aspirin (80 mg/day)

[a] Common bioprosthetic valves: Carpentier-Edwards (bovine and porcine) and Hancock II (porcine). Cryolife, St. Jude, and Medtronic also make porcine bioprostheses.

INR = international normalized ratio; UFH = unfractionated heparin; LMWH = low-molecular-weight heparin; NSR = normal sinus rhythm.

Source: Adapted from *Sixth ACCP Consensus Conference on Antithrombic Therapy: Quick Reference Guide for Clinicians*. American College of Chest Physicians; 2001. With permission.

TABLE 10.6
Definitions Used in Managing Thromboembolic Complications during Pregnancy and Postpartum[3]

Term	Definition
UFH	
Mini-dose	5000 IU sc q12h
Moderate-dose	Adjusted doses, q12h sc, to target an anti-Xa level of 0.1–0.3 IU/ml
Adjusted-dose	Adjusted doses, q12h sc, to target a mid-interval therapeutic APTT
LMWH	
Prophylactic	Dalteparin (5000 IU q24h sc), or enoxaparin (40 mg qd sc), or any qd LMWH adjusted to target a peak (4 h post-dose) anti-Xa level of 0.2 to 0.6 IU/ml
Adjusted-dose	Full, weight-adjusted doses of LMWH, for example, dalteparin (200 IU/kg qd) or enoxaparin (1 mg/kg q12h sc), to achieve an anti-Xa level of approximately 0.5 to 1.2 IU/ml
Postpartum anticoagulants	Warfarin (INR 2–3) given for 4–6 weeks, initially overlapped with UFH or LMWH, until the INR is ≥2.0
Surveillance	Clinical vigilance and aggressive investigation of symptoms suggesting DVT or PE

UFH = unfractionated heparin; APTT = activated partial thromboplastin time; LMWH = low-molecular-weight heparin; INR = international normalized ratio; DVT = deep vein thrombosis; PE = pulmonary embolism; SC = subcutaneous.

Source: *Sixth ACCP Consensus Conference on Antithrombic Therapy: Quick Reference Guide for Clinicians.* American College of Chest Physicians; 2001. With permission.

TABLE 10.7
Pregnant Patients at Increased Risk for VTE[3]

Patient Characteristics	Recommendation
Prior VTE associated with a transient risk factor; no current risk factors (e.g., morbid obesity or strict bed rest)	Surveillance and postpartum anticoagulants
Episode of idiopathic VTE; no current long-term anticoagulant therapy	Options: Surveillance, mini-dose UFH, moderate-dose UFH, or prophylactic LMWH; in addition, postpartum anticoagulants
Episode of VTE; thrombophilia (confirmed laboratory abnormality); no current long-term anticoagulant therapy	Options: Surveillance, mini-dose UFH, moderate-dose UFH, or prophylactic LMWH; in addition, postpartum anticoagulants
No prior VTE; thrombophilia (confirmed laboratory abnormality); no current long-term anticoagulant therapy	Options: Surveillance, mini-dose UFH or prophylactic LMWH; in addition, postpartum anticoagulants; indication for active prophylaxis is strongest in antithrombin-deficient women
≥2 episodes of VTE, and/or long-term anticoagulation (e.g., single episode of VTE, idiopathic or asoociated with thrombophilia)	Options: Adjusted-dose UFH, prophylactic LMWH, or adjusted-dose LMWH; in addition, long-term postpartum anticoagulants

VTE = venous thromboembolism; UFH = unfractionated heparin; LMWH = low-molecular-weight heparin.

Source: *Sixth ACCP Consensus Conference on Antithrombic Therapy: Quick Reference Guide for Clinicians.* American College of Chest Physicians; 2001. With permission.

TABLE 10.8
Treatment of Venous Thromboembolism of Pregnancy[3]

Patient Characteristics	Recommendation
Average risk for recurrent VTE	Adjusted-dose LMWH throughout pregnancy; or IV UFH bolus, followed by continuous infusion to maintain APTT in therapeutic range for ≥ 5 days; then adjusted-dose UFH until delivery
	To avoid unwanted anticoagulation during delivery in women receiving adjusted-dose LMWH or UFH, discontinue heparin therapy 24 h before elective induction of labor
Very high risk for recurrent VTE (e.g., proximal DVT within <2 weeks)	IV UFH, to maintain APTT within therapeutic range; discontinue therapy 4–6 h before expected time of delivery; anticoagulants for ≥ 6 weeks postpartum or ≥ 3 months after VTE
Pregnancy in patients receiving long-term Warfarin	Adjusted-dose UFH or LMWH substituted for Warfarin if pregnancy occurs
Pregnancy in patients with mechanical heart valves	Aggressive adjusted-dose UFH, given q12 h sc throughout pregnancy; mid-interval APTT maintained at ≥ 2 times control levels, or anti-Xa heparin level maintained at 0.35–0.70 IU/ml
	or
	LMWH throughout pregnancy, in doses adjusted according to weight, or as necessary to maintain a 4-h post-injection anti-Xa LMWH level of about 1.0 IU/ml
	or
	UFH or LMWH, as above, until the 13th week; change to Warfarin until the middle of the third trimester, then restart UFH or LMWH therapy until delivery
	In any case, long-term anticoagulation should be resumed postpartum

VTE = venous thromboembolism; LMWH = low-molecular-weight heparin; UFH = unfractionated heparin; APTT = activated partial thromboplastin time; IV = intravenous.

Source: Sixth ACCP Consensus Conference on Antithrombic Therapy: Quick Reference Guide for Clinicians. American College of Chest Physicians; 2001. With permission.

TABLE 10.9
Recommended INR Ranges for Patients Receiving Warfarin[4]

Indication	INR Range
Prophylaxis of venous thrombosis (high-risk surgery)	2.0–3.0
Treatment of venous thrombosis	
Treatment of PE	
Prevention of systemic embolism	
Tissue heart valves	
Acute myocardial infarction	
Valvular heart disease	
Atrial fibrillation	
Mechanical prosthetic valves (high risk)	2.5–3.5
Bileaflet mechanical valve in the aortic position	2.0–3.0
Certain patients with thrombosis and the antiphospholipid syndrome	>2.0–3.0
Recurrent MI	2.5–3.5

INR = international normalized ratio; PE = pulmonary embolism; MI = myocardial infarction.

Source: *Sixth ACCP Consensus Conference on Antithrombic Therapy: Quick Reference Guide for Clinicians*. American College of Chest Physicians; 2001. With permission.

TABLE 10.10
Managing Patients with High INR Values[5]

Situation	Recommendation
INR > therapeutic range but <5.0; no significant bleeding	Lower the dose; or omit the next dose, and resume therapy at a lower dose when the INR is within therapeutic range; if the INR is only slightly above therapeutic range, dose reduction may not be necessary
INR >5.0 but <9.0; no significant bleeding	Omit the next dose or two, monitor INR more frequently, and resume therapy at a lower dose when the INR is within therapeutic range
	Alternatively, omit a dose and give vitamin K (1–2.5 mg po), especially if the patient is at increased risk for bleeding
	Patients requiring more rapid reversal before urgent surgery: vitamin K (2–4 mg PO); if INR remains high at 24 h, an additional dose of vitamin K (1–2 mg po)
INR >9.0; no significant bleeding	Omit Warfarin; give vitamin K (3–5 mg po); closely monitor INR; if the INR is not substantially reduced in 24–48 h, monitor the INR more often, giving additional vitamin K if necessary
	Resume therapy at a lower dose when the INR is within therapeutic range
INR >20; serious bleeding	Omit Warfarin; give prothrombin complex concentrate with vitamin K (10 mg by slow IV infusion); repeat if necessary, depending on the INR
Life-threatening bleeding	Omit Warfarin; give prothrombin complex concentrate with vitamin K (10 mg by slow IV infusion); repeat if necessary, depending on the INR

INR = international normalized ratio.

Source: Sixth ACCP Consensus Conference on Antithrombic Therapy: Quick Reference Guide for Clinicians. American College of Chest Physicians; 2001. With permission.

TABLE 10.11

Managing Warfarin Therapy during and Following Invasive Procedures[5]

Situation	Recommendation
Low risk for thromboembolism (e.g., no VTE for >3 months; atrial fibrillation, without history of stroke; bileaflet mechanical cardiac valve in the aortic position)	Discontinue Warfarin therapy about 4 days before surgery, and allow the INR to return to near-normal levels; if intervention increases a risk for thrombosis, begin short-term low-dose heparin therapy (5000 IU sc) and resume Warfarin therapy
Intermediate risk for thromboembolism (not fitting high-risk or low-risk categories)	Discontinue Warfarin therapy about 4 days before surgery, and allow the INR to fall; about 2 days preoperatively, give either low-dose heparin (5000 IU sc) or a prophylactic dose of LMWH; postoperatively, give low-dose heparin (or LMWH) and Warfarin
High risk for thromboembolism (e.g., VTE within 3 months; history of VTE, mechanical cardiac valve in the mitral position; old-model cardiac valve , i.e., ball/cage)	Discontinue Warfarin about 4 days before surgery and allow the INR to normalize; about 2 days preoperatively, as the INR falls, give full-dose heparin or full-dose LMWH; resume Warfarin postoperatively with full-dose heparin or LMWH until INR is within the target range for 2 consecutive days
	Heparin can be given sc on an outpatient basis, and presurgically, after hospital admission, as a continuous IV infusion, and discontinued 5 h before surgery; alternatively, continue sc heparin or LMWH therapy until 12–24 h before surgery; resume Warfarin postoperatively with full-dose heparin or LMWH until INR is within the target range for 2 consecutive days
Low risk for bleeding	Lower the Warfarin dose 4–5 days before surgery to reach an INR of 1.3–1.5 at the time of surgery; resume Warfarin therapy postoperatively, supplemented, if necessary, with low-dose heparin (5000 IU sc)

TABLE 10.11 (CONTINUED)
Managing Warfarin Therapy during and Following Invasive Procedures[5]

Situation	Recommendation
Dental procedures	Patients at high risk for bleeding discontinue Warfarin therapy; patients not at high risk for bleeding continue Warfarin therapy
Dental procedures, with need to control local bleeding	Administer a mouthwash acid or epsilon aminocaproic acid, without interrupting Warfarin therapy

VTE = venous thromboembolism; INR = international normalized ratio; LMWH = low-molecular-weight heparin.

Source: *Sixth ACCP Consensus Conference on Antithrombic Therapy: Quick Reference Guide for Clinicians*. American College of Chest Physicians; 2001. With permission.

TABLE 10.12
Treatment of Heparin-Induced Thrombocytopenia[6] (HIT)

Situation	Recommendation
Acute HIT with thrombosis	Danaparoid sodium, lepirudin, or argatroban
Acute HIT without thrombosis	Consider danaparoid sodium, lepirudin, or argatroban until the platelet count has recovered
HIT with DVT	Danaparoid sodium or lepirudin; Warfarin should be added once the platelet count is above 100,000

DVT = deep vein thrombosis.

Source: *Sixth ACCP Consensus Conference on Antithrombic Therapy: Quick Reference Guide for Clinicians*. American College of Chest Physicians; 2001. With permission.

TABLE 10.13
Alternative Anticoagulant Drugs[9]

	Danaparoid sodium (Orgaran)	Lepirudin (Refludan)	Argatroban (Acova)	Fondaparinux (Arixtra)
Mechanism of action	Factor Xa and factor IIa inhibitor (ratio >22:1)	Direct thrombin (factor IIa) inhibitor (rDNA)	Direct thrombin (factor IIa) inhibitor (synthetic)	Direct factor Xa inhibitor (synthetic)
FDA-approved indication	Prophylaxis of postoperative DVT in patients undergoing elective hip replacement surgery	Anticoagulation in patients with HIT and associated thrombo-embolic disease	Prevention or treatment of thrombosis in HIT	Prevent DVT in patients undergoing hip fracture surgery, hip replacement surgery or knee replacement surgery
Dose	750 anti-Xa units SQ twice daily beginning 1–4 h preoperatively, and then not sooner than 2 h after surgery; treatment should be continued throughout the period of postoperative care until the risk of DVT has diminished; the average duration of administration in clinical trials was 7–10 days, up to 14 days	0.4 mg/kg (max. 44 mg) slow IV bolus (e.g., over 15 to 20 s), followed by 0.15 mg/kg /hr (max. 16.5 mg/h) IV infusion for 2 to 10 days or longer if clinically needed	2 μg/kg/min IV infusion, adjusted as needed to maintain an aPTT of 1.5–3.0 times control (not to exceed 100 seconds) to a maximum of 10 μg/kg/min	2.5 mg SQ once daily post-operatively; the first dose should be administered 6–8 h following surgical closure, provided hemostasis has been obtained. Usual duration of therapy is 5–9 days

TABLE 10.13 (CONTINUED)
Alternative Anticoagulant Drugs

	Danaparoid sodium (Orgaran)	Lepirudin (Refludan)	Argatroban (Acova)	Fondaparinux (Arixtra)
Antidote	None proved; protamine sulfate is minimally effective	None	None	None
Monitoring	Bleeding complications, periodic CBC, including platelet count	aPTT (target 1.5–2.5 × control) bleeding complications, allergic reactions (cough, bronchospasm, dyspnea, rash, etc.)	Bleeding complications, aPTT	Bleeding complications, platelet count

DVT = deep vein thrombosis; HIT = heparin-induced thrombocytopenia.

Calculation of protamine dosage to reverse heparin[6] (see Figure 10.2):

$$\text{Infusion rate (IU/h)}/42 = \text{total protamine dose (mg)},$$

to be infused slow IV over 10 min

or

$$\text{Bolus dose (IU)}/100 = \text{total protamine dose (mg)}$$

Calculation of protamine dosage to reverse low-molecular-weight heparin[6]: Within 8 h of administering LMWH, use 1 mg/100 anti-Xa units for enoxaparin (1 mg = approximately 100 anti-Xa units). If bleeding continues, a second dose of 0.5 mg/100 anti-Xa units LMWH may be given. Smaller doses are needed beyond 8 h

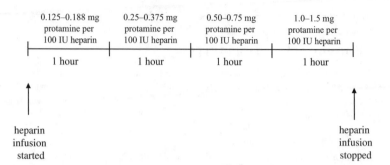

Dosing of protamine for heparin reversal. Based on a 60-min heparin half-life, the dosage of protamine is dictated by the amount of heparin infused in the 4 h prior to heparin discontinuation.

FIGURE 10.2 Reversal of heparin by protamine.

REFERENCES

1. Hyers TM et al. Antithrombotic therapy for venous thromboembolic disease. *Chest.* 2001;119(suppl):176S–193S.
2. Salem DN et al. Antithrombotic therapy in valvular heart disease. *Chest.* 2001;119(suppl):207S–219S.
3. Ginsberg JS, Greer I, Hirsh J. Use of antithrombotic agents during pregnancy. *Chest.* 2001;119(suppl):122S–131S.
4. Hirsh J et al. Oral anticoagulants: mechanism of action, clinical effectiveness, and optimal therapeutic range. *Chest* 2001;119(suppl):8S–21S.
5. Ansell J et al. Managing oral anticoagulant therapy. *Chest.* 2001;119(suppl):22S–38S.
6. Hirsh J et al. Heparin and low-molecular-weight heparin: mechanisms of action, pharmacokinetics, dosing, monitoring, efficacy, and safety. *Chest.* 2001;119(suppl):64S–94S.
7. *Sixth ACCP Consensus Conference on Antithrombotic Therapy: Quick Reference Guide for Clinicians.* American College of Chest Physicians; Northbrook, IL. 2001.
8. Stein PD, Alpert JS, Bussey HI, Dalen JE, Turpie AGG. Antithrombotic therapy in patients with mechanical and biological prosthetic heart valves. Chest 2001;119(suppl.):220S–227S.
9. Prescribing information.

11 Endocarditis: Prophylaxis and Treatment

Judy W.M. Cheng

CONTENTS

TABLE 11.1
Cardiac Conditions Associated with Endocarditis[1-21]

Endocarditis Prophylaxis Recommended

High-risk category

Prosthetic cardiac valves, including bioprosthetic and homograft valves

Previous bacterial endocarditis

Complex cyanotic congenital heart disease (e.g., single ventricle states, transposition of the great arteries, tetralogy of Fallot)

Surgically constructed systemic pulmonary shunts or conduits

Moderate-risk category

Most other congenital cardiac malformations (other than above and below)

Acquired valvular dysfunction (e.g., rheumatic heart disease)

Hypertrophic cardiomyopathy

Mitral valve prolapse with valvular regurgitation and/or thickened leaflets

Endocarditis Prophylaxis Not Recommended

Negligible-risk category (no greater risk than the general population)

Isolated secundum atrial septal defect

Surgical repair of atrial septal defect, ventricular septal defect, or patent ductus arteriosus (without residual beyond 6 months)

Previous coronary artery bypass graft surgery

Mitral valve prolapse without valvular regurgitation

Physiologic, functional, or innocent heart murmurs

Previous Kawasaki disease without valvular dysfunction

Previous rheumatic fever without valvular dysfunction

Cardiac pacemakers (intravascular and epicardial) and implanted defibrillators

Source: American Heart Association. Publ 71-0117;1997. With permission.

TABLE 11.2
Dental Procedures and Endocarditis Prophylaxis[21-29]

Endocarditis Prophylaxis Recommended[a]

Dental extractions

Periodontal procedures including surgery, scaling and root planing, probing, and recall maintenance

Dental implant placement and reimplantation of avulsed teeth

Endodontic (root canal) instrumentation or surgery only beyond the apex

Subgingival placement of antibiotic fibers or strips

Initial placement of orthodontic bands but not brackets

Intraligamentary local anesthetic injections

Prophylactic cleaning of teeth or implants where bleeding is anticipated

Endocarditis Prophylaxis Not Recommended

Restorative dentistry[b] (operative and prosthodontic) with or without retraction cord[c]

Local anesthetic injections (nonintraligamentary)

Intracanal endodontic treatment; postplacement and buildup

Placement of rubber dams

Postoperative suture removal

Placement of removable prosthodontic or orthodontic appliances

Taking of oral impressions

Fluoride treatments

Taking of oral radiographs

Orthodontic appliance adjustment

Shedding of primary teeth

[a] Prophylaxis is recommended for patients with high- and moderate-risk cardiac conditions.

[b] This includes restoration of decayed teeth (filling cavities) and replacement of missing teeth.

[c] Clinical judgment may indicate antibiotic use in selected circumstances that may create significant bleeding.

Source: American Heart Association. Publ 71-0117;1997. With permission.

TABLE 11.3
Other Procedures and Endocarditis Prophylaxis[30-53]

Endocarditis Prophylaxis Recommended

Respiratory tract
  Tonsillectomy and/or adenoidectomy
  Surgical operations that involve respiratory mucosa
  Bronchoscopy with a rigid bronchoscope
Gastrointestinal tract[a]
  Sclerotherapy for esophageal varices
  Esophageal stricture dilation
  Endoscopic retrograde cholangiography with biliary obstruction
  Biliary tract surgery
  Surgical operations that involve intestinal mucosa
Genitourinary tract
  Prostatic surgery
  Cystoscopy
  Urethral dilation

Endocarditis Prophylaxis Not Recommended

Respiratory tract
  Endotracheal intubation
  Bronchoscopy with a flexible bronchoscope, with or without biopsy[b]
  Tympanostomy tube insertion
Gastrointestinal tract
  Transesophageal echocardiography[b]
  Endoscopy with or without gastrointestinal biopsy[b]
Genitourinary tract
  Vaginal hysterectomy[b]
  Vaginal delivery[b]
  Cesarean section
  In uninfected tissue:
    Urethral catheterization
    Uterine dilatation and curettage
    Therapeutic abortion
    Sterilization procedures
    Insertion or removal of intrauterine devices

TABLE 11.3 (CONTINUED)
Other Procedures and Endocarditis Prophylaxis[30-53]

Other
    Cardiac catheterization, including balloon angioplasty
    Implanted cardiac pacemakers, implanted defibrillators, and coronary stents
    Incision or biopsy of surgically scrubbed skin
    Circumcision

[a] Prophylaxis is recommended for high-risk patients; it is optional for medium-risk patients.

[b] Prophylaxis is optional for high-risk patients.

Source: American Heart Association. Publ 71-0117;1997. With permission.

TABLE 11.4

Prophylactic Regimens for Dental, Oral, Respiratory Tract, or Esophageal Procedures[21,54]

Situation	Agent[a]	Regimen
Standard general prophylaxis	Amoxicillin	Adults: 2.0 g; children: 50 mg/kg orally 1 h before procedure
Unable to take oral medications	Ampicillin	Adults: 2.0 g IM or IV; children: 50 mg/kg IM or IV within 30 min before procedure
Allergic to penicillin	Clindamycin, or	Adults: 600 mg; children: 20 mg/kg orally 1 h before procedure
	Cephalexin,[b] or	Adults: 2.0 g; children: 50 mg/kg orally 1 h before procedure
	Cefadroxil,[b] or	Adults: 2.0 g; children: 50 mg/kg orally 1 h before procedure
	Azithromycin, or	500 mg; children: 15 mg/kg orally 1 h before procedure
	Clarithromycin	Adults: 500 mg; children: 15 mg/kg orally 1 h before procedure
Allergic to penicillin and unable to take oral medications	Clindamycin, or	Adults: 600 mg; children: 20 mg/kg IV within 30 min before procedure
	Cefazolin[b]	Adults: 1.0 g; children: 25 mg/kg IM or IV within 30 min before procedure

IM = intramuscularly; IV = intravenously.

[a] Total children's dose should not exceed adult dose.

[b] Cephalosporins should not be used in individuals with immediate-type hypersensitivity reaction (urticaria, angioedema, or anaphylaxis) to penicillins.

Source: American Heart Association. Publ 71-0117;1997. With permission.

TABLE 11.5

Prophylactic Regimens for Genitourinary/Gastrointestinal (Excluding Esophageal) Procedures[21]

Situation	Agents[a]	Regimen[b]
High-risk patients	Ampicillin plus gentamicin	Adults: ampicillin 2.0 g IM or IV plus gentamicin 1.5 mg/kg (not to exceed 120 mg) within 30 min of starting procedure; 6 h later, ampicillin 1 g IM/IV or amoxicillin 1 g orally Children: ampicillin 50 mg/kg IM or IV (not to exceed 2.0 g) plus gentamicin 1.5 mg/kg within 30 min of starting the procedure; 6 h later, ampicillin 25 mg/kg IM/IV or amoxicillin 25 mg/kg orally
High-risk patients allergic to ampicillin/amoxicillin	Vancomycin plus gentamicin	Adults: vancomycin 1.0 g IV over 1–2 h plus gentamicin 1.5 mg/kg IV/IM (not to exceed 120 mg); complete injection/infusion within 30 min of starting procedure Children: vancomycin 20 mg/kg IV over 1–2 h plus gentamicin 1.5 mg/kg IV/IM; complete injection/infusion within 30 min of starting procedure
Moderate-risk patients	Amoxicillin or ampicillin	Adults: amoxicillin 2.0 g orally 1 h before procedure, or ampicillin 2.0 g IM/IV within 30 min of starting procedure Children: amoxicillin 50 mg/kg orally 1 h before procedure, or ampicillin 50 mg/kg IM/IV within 30 min of starting procedure

TABLE 11.5 (CONTINUED)
Prophylactic Regimens for Genitourinary/Gastrointestinal
(Excluding Esophageal) Procedures[21]

Situation	Agents[a]	Regimen[b]
Moderate-risk patients allergic to ampicillin/amoxicillin	Vancomycin	Adults: vancomycin 1.0 g IV over 1–2 h; complete infusion within 30 min of starting procedure Children: vancomycin 20 mg/kg IV over 1–2 h; complete infusion within 30 min of starting procedure

IM = intramuscularly; IV = intravenously.

[a] Total children's dose should not exceed adult dose.

[b] No second dose of vancomycin or gentamicin is recommended.

Source: American Heart Association. Publ 71-0117;1997. With permission.

TABLE 11.6
Treatment of Confirmed Infective Endocarditis

Diagnosis and Etiologies	Regimen	Duration of treatment	Comments
Native Valve **(patients with congenital heart disease including mitral valve prolapse)[55,56]**			
Strep viridans *Strep bovis* (Pen G MIC <0.1 mg/l)	Primary: Penicillin G 12–18 million units daily IV divided into q4 h	4 weeks	Target gentamicin level: peak 3 mg/l, trough <1 mg/l
	Alternative (if Penicillin Allergic): Ceftriaxone 2 g qd IV + gentamicin 1 mg/kg IV q8 h	2 weeks	Target vancomycin level: peak 20–50 mg/dl, trough 5–12 mg/l
	Vancomycin 30 mg/kg/ day in 2 divided doses	4 weeks	
Strep viridans *Strep bovis* (Pen G MIC >0.1 mg/l but <0.5 mg/l)	Primary: Penicillin G 18 million units daily IV divided into q4 h + gentamicin 1 mg/kg IV q8 h	4 weeks (Pen G), 2 weeks (gentamicin)	Target gentamicin level: peak 3 mg/l, trough <1 mg/l
	Alternative (if penicillin allergic): Vancomycin 30 mg/kg/ day in 2 divided doses (if allergic to penicillin) + gentamicin 1 mg/kg IV q8 h	4 weeks	Target vancomycin level: peak 20–50 mg/dl, trough 5–12 mg/l
Strep viridans *Strep bovis* (Pen G MIC >1 mg/l) *Enterococci* Susceptable to Pen G, Vancomycin, and gentamicin	Primary: Penicillin G 18–30 million units daily IV divided into q4 h + gentamicin 1 mg/kg IV q8 h	4–6 weeks	4 weeks if symptoms <3 months, 6 weeks if symptoms >3 months
	Ampicillin 12 g/day divided into q4 h + gentamicin 1 mg/kg IV q8 h	4–6 weeks	Target gentamicin level: peak 3 mg/l, trough <1 mg/l

TABLE 11.6 (CONTINUED)
Treatment of Confirmed Infective Endocarditis

Diagnosis and Etiologies	Regimen	Duration of treatment	Comments
	Alternative (if penicillin allergic): Vancomycin 30 mg/kg/day in 2 divided doses (if allergic to penicillin)	4–6 weeks	Target vancomycin level: peak 20–50 mg/dl, trough 5–12 mg/l
Enterococci MIC streptomycin >2000 mg/l MIC gentamicin >500–2000 mg/l No resistance to penicillin	Primary: Penicillin G 18–30 million units daily IV divided into q4 h Ampicillin 12 g/day divided into q4 h	8–12 weeks	
Enterococci Beta-lactamase test production test is positive but no gentamicin resistance	Primary: Ampicillin/Salbactam 3 g IV q6 h + gentamicin 1 mg/kg IV q8 h	4–6 weeks	
	Alternative: Ampicillin/Sulbactam 3 g IV q6 h + vancomycin 30 mg/kg/day in 2 divided doses	4–6 weeks	
Enterococci Beta-lactamase test production test is negative but no gentamicin resistance	Vancomycin 30 mg/kg /day in 2 divided doses + gentamicin 1 mg/kg IV q8 h	4–6 weeks	

TABLE 11.6 (CONTINUED)
Treatment of Confirmed Infective Endocarditis

Diagnosis and Etiologies	Regimen	Duration of treatment	Comments
Enterococci Resistant to all penicillin, ampicillin, gentamicin	Quinupristin/dalfopristin (Synercid) (for *E. faecium*, not effective for *E. fecalis*) or Linezolid (no reliable effective treatment)		
Staphylococci Methicillin sensitive	Primary: Nafcillin 2 g q4 h IV + gentamicin 1 mg/kg IV q8 h	Nafcillin 4–6 weeks Gentamicin 3–5 days (2 weeks if tricuspid valve is involved)	
	Alternative: Cefazolin 2 g IV q8 h + gentamicin 1 mg/kg IV q8 h Vancomycin 30 mg/kg/day in 2 divided doses	Cefazolin 4–6 weeks Gentamicin 3–5 days 4–6 weeks	
Methicllin resistant *Staph aureus*	Vancomycin 30 mg/kg/day in 2 divided doses	4–6 weeks	

TABLE 11.6 (CONTINUED)
Treatment of Confirmed Infective Endocarditis

Diagnosis and Etiologies	Regimen	Duration of treatment	Comments
Slow growing fastidious Gram negative bacilli (HACEK group including *H. parainfluenza, H. aphrophilus, A. actinomycetemocomitans, C. hominis, E. corrodens, K. kingae*)	Primary: Ceftriaxone 2 g qd IV Alternative: Ampicillin 12 g daily IV given q4 h + gentamicin 1 mg/kg IV q8 h	4 weeks 4 weeks	

Prosthetic Valve

Diagnosis and Etiologies	Regimen	Duration of treatment	Comments
Strep viridans *Strep bovis* (Pen G MIC <0.1 mg/l)	Primary: Penicillin G 12–18 million units daily IV divided into q4 h Alternative (if penicillin allergic): Ceftriaxone 2 g qd IV + gentamicin 1 mg/kg IV q8 h Vancomycin 30 mg/kg/ day in 2 divided doses	2–4 weeks 2 weeks 4 weeks	Target gentamicin level: peak 3 mg/l, trough <1 mg/l Target vancomycin level: peak 20–50 mg/dl, trough 5–12 mg/l
Strep viridans *Strep bovis* (Pen G MIC >0.1 mg/l but < 0.5 mg/l)	Primary: Penicillin G 18 million units daily IV divided into q4 h + gentamicin 1 mg/kg IV q8 h Alternative (if penicillin allergic): Vancomycin 30 mg/kg/day in 2 divided doses (if allergic to penicillin)	4 weeks (Pen G), 2 weeks (gentamicin) 4 weeks	Target gentamicin level: peak 3 mg/l, trough <1 mg/l Target vancomycin level: peak 20–50 mg/dl, trough 5–12 mg/l

TABLE 11.6 (CONTINUED)
Treatment of Confirmed Infective Endocarditis

Diagnosis and Etiologies	Regimen	Duration of treatment	Comments
Strep viridans *Strep bovis* (Pen G MIC >1 mg/l) *Enterococci* susceptable to Pen G, vancomycin and gentamicin	Primary: Penicillin G 18–30 million units daily IV divided into q4 h + gentamicin 1 mg/kg IV q8 h	4–6 weeks	4 weeks if symptoms <3 months, 6 weeks if symptoms >3 months
	Ampicillin 12 g/day divided into q4 h + gentamicin 1 mg/kg IV q8 h	4–6 weeks	Target gentamicin level: peak 3 mg/l, trough <1 mg/l
	Alternative (if penicillin allergic): Vancomycin 30 mg/kg/day in 2 divided doses (if allergic to penicillin) + gentamicin 1 mg/kg IV q8 h	4–6 weeks	Target vancomycin level: peak 20–50 mg/dl, trough 5–12 mg/l
Enterococci MIC Streptomycin >2000 mg/l MIC gentamicin >500–2000 mg/l No resistant to penicillin	Primary: Penicillin G 18–30 million units daily IV divided into q4 h + gentamicin 1 mg/kg IV q8 h Ampicillin 12 g/day divided into q4 h	8–12 weeks	
Enterococci Beta-lactamase production test is positive and no gentamicin resistance	Primary: Ampicillin/Salbactam 3 g IV q6 h + gentamicin 1 mg/kg IV q8 h Alternative: Ampicillin/Salbactam 3 g IV q6 h + vancomycin 30 mg/kg/day in 2 divided doses	4–6 weeks 4–6 weeks	

TABLE 11.6 (CONTINUED)
Treatment of Confirmed Infective Endocarditis

Diagnosis and Etiologies	Regimen	Duration of treatment	Comments
Enterococci Beta-lactamase production test is negative but no gentamicin resistance	Vancomycin 30 mg/kg/day in 2 divided doses + gentamicin 1 mg/kg IV q8 h	4–6 weeks	
Enterococci Resistant to all penicillin, ampicillin, gentamicin, vancomycin	Quinupristin/dalfopristin (Synercid) (for *E. faecium*, not effective for *E. fecalis*) or Linezolid (no reliable effective treatment)		
Methicllin-sensitive *S. aureus*	Naficillin 2 g IV q4 h + rifampin 300 mg po q8 h + gentamicin 1 mg/kg IV q8 h	Nafcillin and rifampin, 6 weeks; gentamicin, 14 days	
	Vancomycin 30 mg/kg/day in 2 divided doses + rifampin 300 mg po q8 h + gentamicin 1 mg/kg IV q8 h	Vancomycin and rifampin, 6 weeks; gentamicin 14 days	

TABLE 11.6 (CONTINUED)
Treatment of Confirmed Infective Endocarditis

Diagnosis and Etiologies	Regimen	Duration of treatment	Comments
Enterobacteriaceae or *Pseudomonas aeuroginosa*	Antipseudomonal penicillin or antipseudomonal 3rd generation cephalosporins or 4th generation cephalosporins (e.g., Piperacillin 18 g/day IV dividied into q6 h) + tobramycin 5–8 mg/kg//day IV given q8 h	6 weeks	Rarely effective, valve replacement usually necessary

Source: American Heart Association. Publ 71-0117;1997. With permission.

REFERENCES

1. Steckelberg JM, Wilson WR. Risk factors for infective endocarditis. *Infect Dis Clin North Am.* 1993;7:9–19.
2. Saiman L, Prince A, Gersony WM. Pediatric infective endocarditis in the modern era. *J Pediatr.* 1993;122:847–853.
3. Gersony WM et al. Bacterial endocarditis in patients with aortic stenosis, pulmonary stenosis, or ventricular septal defect. *Circulation.* 1993;87(suppl I):I-121–I-126.
4. Prabhu SD, O'Rourke RA. Mitral valve prolapse. In: Braunwald E, series ed, Rahimtoola SH, volume ed. *Atlas of Heart Diseases: Valvular Heart Disease*: Vol XI. St. Louis, MO: Mosby-Year Book; 1997:10.1–10.18.
5. Boudoulas H, Wooley CF. Mitral valve prolapse. In: Emmanouilides GC et al. eds. *Moss and Adams Heart Disease in Infants, Children, and Adolescents Including the Fetus and Young Adult.* 5th ed. Baltimore, MD: Williams & Wilkins; 1995:1063–1086.
6. Carabello BA. Mitral valve disease. *Curr Probl Cardiol.* 1993;7:423–478.
7. Devereux RB et al. Complications of mitral valve prolapse: disproportionate occurrence in men and older patients. *Am J Med.* 1986;81:751–758.

8. Danchin N et al. Mitral valve prolapse as a risk factor for infective endocarditis. *Lancet.* 1989;1:743–745.

9. MacMahon SW et al. Mitral valve prolapse and infective endocarditis. *Am Heart J.* 1987;113:1291–1298.

10. Marks AR et al. Identification of high-risk and low-risk subgroups of patients with mitral-valve prolapse. *New Engl J Med.* 1989;320:1031–1036.

11. Devereux RB et al. Cost-effectiveness of infective endocarditis prophylaxis for mitral valve prolapse with or without a mitral regurgitant murmur. *Am J Cardiol.* 1994;74:1024–1029.

12. Zuppiroli A et al. Natural history of mitral valve prolapse. *Am J Cardiol.* 1995;75:1028–1032.

13. Wooley CF et al. The floppy, myxomatous mitral valve, mitral valve prolapse, and mitral regurgitation. *Prog Cardiovasc Dis.* 1991;33:397–433.

14. Morales AR et al. Myxoid heart disease: an assessment of extravalvular cardiac pathology in severe mitral valve prolapse. *Hum Pathol.* 1992;23:129–137.

15. Weissman N et al. In vivo mitral valve morphology and motion in mitral valve prolapse. *Am J Cardiol.* 1994;73:1080–1088.

16. Nishimura RA et al. Echocardiographically documented mitral-valve prolapse. *New Engl J Med.* 1985;313:1305–1309.

17. McKinsey DS, Ratts TE, Bisno AL. Underlying cardiac lesions in adults with infective endocarditis. *Am J Med.* 1987;82:681–688.

18. Devereux RB, Kramer-Fox R, Kligfield P. Mitral valve prolapse: causes, clinical manifestations, and management. *Ann Intern Med.* 1989;111:305–317.

19. Stoddard MF et al. Exercise-induced mitral regurgitation is a predictor of morbid events in subjects with mitral valve prolapse. *J Am Coll Cardiol.* 1995;25:693–699.

20. Awadallah SM et al. The changing pattern of infective endocarditis in childhood. *Am J Cardiol.* 1991;68:90–94.

21. Durack DT. Prevention of infective endocarditis. *New Engl J Med.* 1995;332:38–44.

22. Pallasch TJ, Slots J. Antibiotic prophylaxis and the medically compromised patient. *Periodontol.* 2000. 1996;10:107–138.

23. Bender IB, Naidorf IJ, Garvey GJ. Bacterial endocarditis: a consideration for physicians and dentists. *J Am Dent Assoc.* 1984;109:415–420.

24. Guntheroth WG. How important are dental procedures as a cause of infective endocarditis? *Am J Cardiol.* 1984;54:797–801.

25. Roman AR, App GR. Bacteremia, a result from oral irrigation in subjects with gingivitis. *J Periodontol.* 1971;42:757–760.

26. Felix JE, Rosen S, App GR. Detection of bacteremia after the use of oral irrigation device on subjects with periodontitis. *J Periodontol.* 1971;42:785–787.

27. Hunter KD et al. Bacteremia and tissue damage resulting from air polishing. *Br Dent J.* 1989;167:275–277.

28. Berger SA et al. Bacteremia after use of an oral irrigating device. *Ann Intern Med.* 1974;80:510–511.

29. Niv Y, Bat L, Motro M. Bacterial endocarditis after Hurst bougienage in a patient with a benign esophageal stricture and mitral valve prolapse. *Gastrointest Endosc.* 1985;31:265–267.

30. Rodriguez W, Levine J. Enterococcal endocarditis following flexible sigmoidoscopy. *West J Med.* 1984;140:951–953.

31. Rigilano J, et al. Enterococcal endocarditis following sigmoidoscopy and mitral valve prolapse. *Arch Intern Med.* 1984;144:850–851.

32. Pritchard T et al. Prosthetic valve endocarditis due to *Cardiobacterium hominis* occurring after upper gastrointestinal endoscopy. *Am J Med.* 1991;90:516–518.

33. Watanakunakorn C. *Streptococcus bovis* endocarditis associated with villous adenoma following colonoscopy. *Am Heart J.* 1988;116:1115–1116.

34. Baskin G. Prosthetic endocarditis after endoscopic variceal sclerotherapy: a failure of antibiotic prophylaxis. *Am J Gastroenterol.* 1989;84:311–312.

35. Yin T, Dellipiani A. Bacterial endocarditis after Hurst bougienage in a patient with a benign esophageal stricture. *Endoscopy.* 1983;15:27–28.

36. Norfleet R. Infectious endocarditis after fiberoptic sigmoidoscopy. *J Clin Gastroenterol.* 1991;13:448–451.

37. Logan R, Hastings J. Bacterial endocarditis: a complication of gastroscopy. *Br Med J.* 1988;296:1107.

38. Botoman V, Surawicz C. Bacteremia with gastrointestinal endoscopic procedures. *Gastrointest Endosc.* 1986;32:342–346.

39. Bryne W et al. Bacteremia in children following upper gastrointestinal endoscopy or colonoscopy. *J Pediatr Gastroenterol Nutr.* 1982;1:551–553.

40. Shull H et al. Bacteremia with upper gastrointestinal endoscopy. *Ann Intern Med.* 1975;83:212–214.

41. Low D et al. Prospective assessment of risk of bacteremia with colonoscopy and polypectomy. *Dig Dis Sci.* 1987;32:1239–1243.

42. Low D et al. Risk of bacteremia with endoscopic sphincterotomy. *Can J Surg.* 1987;30:421–423.

43. Raines DR et al. The occurrence of bacteremia after oesophageal dilatation. *Gastrointest Endosc.* 1975;22:86–87.

44. Welsh JD et al. Bacteremia associated with esophageal dilation. *J Clin Gastroenterol.* 1983;5:109–112.

45. Yin TP, Dellipiana AW. The incidence of bacteremia after outpatient Hurst bougienage in the management of benign esophageal stricture. *Endoscopy.* 1983;31:265–267.

46. Stephenson PM et al. Bacteraemia following oesophageal dilatation and oesophagogastroscopy. *Aust N Z J Med.* 1977;7:32–35.

47. Ho H, Zuckerman M, Wassem C. A prospective controlled study of the risk of bacteremia in emergency sclerotherapy of esophageal varices [Abstract]. *Gastroenterology.* 1991;101:1642–1648.

48. Cohen L et al. Bacteremia after endoscopic injection sclerosis. *Gastrointest Endosc.* 1983;29:198–200.

49. Tseng C et al. Bacteremia after endoscopic band ligation of esophageal varices. *Gastrointest Endosc.* 1992;38:336–337.

50. Sullivan N et al. Clinical aspects of bacteremia after manipulation of the genitourinary tract. *J Infect Dis.* 1973;127:49–55.

51. Sugrue D et al. Antibiotic prophylaxis against infective endocarditis after normal delivery: is it necessary[Abstract]? *Br Heart J.* 1980;44:499–502.

52. Child JS. Risks for and prevention of infective endocarditis. In: Child JS, ed. *Cardiology Clinics — Diagnosis and Management of Infective Endocarditis.* Philadelphia: WB Saunders; 1996;14:327–343.

53. Dajani AS, Bawdon RE, Berry MC. Oral amoxicillin as prophylaxis for endocarditis: what is the optimal dose? *Clin Infect Dis.* 1994;18:157–160.

54. Fluckiger U et al. Role of amoxicillin serum levels for successful prophylaxis of experimental endocarditis due to tolerant *streptococci. J Infect Dis.* 1994;169:397–400.

55. Wilson WR et al. Antibiotic treatment of adults with infective endocarditis due to *streptococci, enterococci, staphylococci,* and HACEK microorganisms. American Heart Association. *J Am Med Assoc.* 1995;274(21):1706–1713.

56. Bayer AS et al. Diagnosis and management of infective endocarditis and its complications. *Circulation.* 1998;98:2936–2948.

57. Dajani AS et al. Prevention of bacterial endocarditis: recommendations by the American Heart Association. *Circulation.* 1997;96:358–366.

12 Medication-Induced Cardiovascular Side Effects

Cynthia A. Sanoski

CONTENTS

TABLE 12.1
Drugs That Cause QT Interval Prolongation and/or Torsades de Pointes

Anesthetic agents
  Enflurane[1]
  Isoflurane[1,2]
  Halothane[1,3]
Antianginals
  Bepridil[4-6]
Antiarrhythmics
  Amiodarone[7-14]
  Disopyramide[15-18]
  Dofetilide[19-21]
  Ibutilide[22]
  Procainamide[23,24]
  Quinidine[25,26]
  Sotalol[7,19,27-30]
Antidepressants
  Amitriptyline[31,32]
  Desipramine[33]
  Doxepin[34-36]
  Imipramine[37]
  Nortriptyline
Antimalarial
  Halofantrine[38,39]
Antimicrobials
  Clarithromycin[40-42]
  Erythromycin[43-48]
  Fluconazole[49]
  Gatifloxacin[50]
  Itraconazole[51]
  Ketoconzole[52]
  Levofloxacin[53]
  Moxifloxacin[50,54,55]
  Pentamidine[56-62]
  Sparfloxacin[50,63,64]
  Trimethoprim-sulfamethoxazole[65,66]

Antineoplastic agents
  Arsenic trioxide[67-71]
  Tamoxifen[72,73]
Antipsychotics
  Chlorpromazine[74,75]
  Haloperidol[76-82]
  Mesoridazine[83]
  Pimozide[84]
  Quetiapine[85,86]
  Thioridazine[83,87-89]
Diuretics
  Indapamide[90]
Immunosuppressants
  Tacrolimus[91-93]
Sedatives/hypnotics
  Droperidol[79,89,94,95]

TABLE 12.2
Cardiovascular Side Effects of Psychiatric Medications

Tricyclic Antidepressants (TCAs)

Amitriptyline
 Hypotension
 Orthostatic hypotension
 Tachycardia
 QT interval prolongation
 Ventricular arrhythmias

Clomipramine
 Hypotension
 Ventricular arrhythmias

Desipramine
 Hypotension
 QT interval prolongation
 Ventricular arrhythmias

Doxepin
 Hypotension
 QT interval prolongation
 Ventricular arrhythmias

Imipramine
 Orthostatic hypotension
 Tachycardia
 QT interval prolongation
 Ventricular arrhythmias

Nortriptyline
 Orthostatic hypotension
 Tachycardia
 QT interval prolongation
 Ventricular arrhythmias

Monoamine Oxidase Inhibitors (MAOIs)

Phenelzine
 Orthostatic hypotension
 Tachycardia
 Peripheral edema
 Hypertensive crisis (if tyramine-containing foods are concomitantly ingested)

TABLE 12.2 (CONTINUED)
Cardiovascular Side Effects of Psychiatric Medications

Tranylcypromine
Orthostatic hypotension
Hypertensive crisis (if tyramine-containing foods are concomitantly ingested)

Second-Generation Antidepressants

Buproprion
Tachycardia
Hypotension
Palpitations

Selective Serotonic Reuptake Inhibitors (SSRIs)

Fluoxetine
Hypertension
Palpitations
Fluvoxamine
Palpitations
Paroxetine
Palpitations
Orthostatic hypotension
Sertraline
Palpitations

Other Antidepressants

Venlafaxine
Hypertension
Tachycardia
Orthostatic hypotension
Mirtazapine
Hypertension
Peripheral edema
Nefazodone
Orthostatic hypotension

Antipsychotic Agents

Chlorpromazine
Hypotension
Orthostatic hypotension
Tachycardia

TABLE 12.2 (CONTINUED)
Cardiovascular Side Effects of Psychiatric Medications

QT interval prolongation
Ventricular arrhythmias
Clozapine
Tachycardia
Hypotension
Orthostatic hypotension
Hypertension
Haloperidol
Orthostatic hypotension
QT interval prolongation
Ventricular arrhythmias
Mesoridazine
Hypotension
Orthostatic hypotension
Perphenazine
Hypotension
Orthostatic hypotension
Pimozide
Tachycardia
Orthostatic hypotension
QT interval prolongation
Ventricular arrhythmias
Risperidone
Orthostatic hypotension
Tachycardia
Thioridazine
Hypotension
Orthostatic hypotension
QT interval prolongation
Ventricular arrhythmias
Thiothixine
Hypotension
Orthostatic hypotension

TABLE 12.3
Potential Drug Interactions with Warfarin

Drugs That May Increase Warfarin Effects (May Increase PT/INR)	Drugs That May Decrease Warfarin Effects (May Decrease PT/INR)
Acetaminophen	Alcohol
Alcohol	Aminoglutethimide
Allopurinol	Amobarbital
Aminosalicylic acid	Antipyrine
Amiodarone	Azathiprine
Androgens	Butabarbital
Aspirin	Butalbital
Atorvastatin	Carbamazepine
Azithromycin	Cholestyramine
Cefoperazone	Chlordiazepoxide
Cefamandole	Chlorthalidone
Cefotetan	Colestipol
Chloral hydrate	Cyclophosphamide
Chloramphenicol	Cyclosporine
Chlorpropamide	Dicloxacillin
Cimetidine	Disopyramide
Ciprofloxacin	Haloperidol
Clarithromycin	Meprobamate
Clopidogrel	6-Mercaptopurine
Danazol	Methimiazole
Dextran	Mitotane
Diazoxide	Nafcillin
Diclofenac	Oral contraceptives
Diflunisal	Pentobarbital
Disulfuram	Phenobarbital
Doxycycline	Phenytoin
Erythromycin	Primidone
Ethacrynic acid	Propylthiouracil
Etoposide	Secobarbital
Fluconazole	Sucralfate
Fluorouracil	Trazodone
Fluoxetine	
Fluvoxamine	
Gemfibrozil	

TABLE 12.3 (CONTINUED)
Potential Drug Interactions with Warfarin

**Drugs That May Increase Warfarin
Effects (May Increase PT/INR)**

Glucagon
Glyburide
Griseofulvin
Heparin
Ibuprofen
Ifosfamide
Indomethacin
Influenza vaccine
Isoniazid
Itraconazole
Ketoconazole
Ketoprofen
Ketorolac
Levamisole
Levothyroxine
Liothyronine
Lovastatin
Methyldopa
Metronidazole
Methimazole
Miconazole
Nalidixic acid
Naproxen
Neomycin
Ofloxacin
Omeprazole
Paroxetine
Penicillin
Pentoxyfylline
Phenytoin
Piperacillin
Piroxicam
Prednisone
Propranolol

TABLE 12.3 (CONTINUED)
Potential Drug Interactions with Warfarin

Drugs That May Increase Warfarin Effects (May Increase PT/INR)

Propafenone
Propoxyphene
Quinidine
Quinine
Ranitidine
Sertraline
Simvastatin
Sulfamethoxazole
Sulfisoxazole
Sulindac
Tamoxifen
Tetracycline
Thyroid hormone
Ticarcillin
Ticlopidine
Tricyclic antidepressants
Trimethoprim-sulfamethoxazole
Valproic acid
Vitamin E

Source: Adapted from Harder S. Thurmann P. *Clin Pharmacokinet*. 1996;30: 416–444; Wells PS et al. *Ann Intern Med*. 1994. 1994;121:676–683; Freedman MD, Olatidoye AG. *Drug Saf*. 1994;10:381–394.

TABLE 12.4
Potential Cardiovascular Side Effects of Chemotherapeutic Agents

Chemotherapeutic Agent	Cardiovascular Adverse Effects

Anthracyclines (doxorubicin, daunorubicin, idarubicin)[a]	Acute effects (occur during and within hours after administration)[99,100]
	  Supraventricular arrhythmias
	  Ventricular ectopy
	
	Subacute effects (occur within days or weeks after administration)[101,102]
	  Myocarditis
	  Pericarditis
	
	Chronic effects (occur weeks or months after administration)[103-105]
	  Cardiomyopathy (especially with cumulative doses >550 mg/m² of doxorubicin)
	
	Risk Factors for Cardiotoxicity:
	  Cumulative dose (>550 mg/m² with doxorubicin)
	  Schedule of administration (toxicity less with administration of more frequent lower doses)
	  Prior mediastinal radiation
	  Underlying cardiac disease
	  Age (children and elderly people more likely to experience cardiotoxicity with lower doses)

Mitoxantrone	Cardiotoxic effects similar to anthracyclines (appears to be less cardiotoxic than anthracyclines)[107,108]
	
	Risk Factors for Cardiotoxicity:
	  Prior mediastinal radiation
	  Underlying cardiac disease
	  Prior anthracycline (doxorubicin) exposure

Bleomycin	Pericarditis (associated with ST-segment elevation)[109,110]

TABLE 12.4 (CONTINUED)
Potential Cardiovascular Side Effects of Chemotherapeutic Agents

Chemotherapeutic Agent	Cardiovascular Adverse Effects
Dactinomycin	Pericarditis[111,112]
Cyclophosphamide	Transient electrocardiographic changes
	Asymptomatic elevation of cardiac enzymes
	Pericarditis
	Cardiotoxic effects are rare with standard doses and are more likely to occur when very high doses are used (total dose >100 mg/kg)[113,114]
Ifosfamide	Cardiomyopathy (risk may be increased when higher doses are used or if administered concomitantly with doxorubicin)[115,116]
Cisplatin	Transient electrocardiographic changes (e.g., ST-T segment abnormalities)[117]
	Supraventricular arrhythmias[118]
	Conduction abnormalities (e.g., bundle-branch blocks)
	Transient coronary ischemia
Mechlorethamine	Sinus tachycardia (risk may be increased when higher doses are used)[119]
5-Fluorouracil	Angina pectoris[120]
	Myocardial infarction[121]
	Supraventricular/ventricular arrhythmias[122]
Vincristine	Myocardial infarction[123,124]

[a] Idarubicin may produce less cardiotoxic effects than doxorubicin and daunorubicin.[106]

REFERENCES

1. Schmeling WT et al. Prolongation of the QT interval by enflurane, isoflurane, and halothane in humans. *Anesth Analg.* 1991;72:137–144.
2. Michaloudis D et al. Anaesthesia and the QT interval in humans: effects of halothane and isoflurane in premedicated children. *Eur J Anaesthesiol.* 1998;15:623–628.
3. Weissenburger J, Nesterenko VV, Antelevitch C. Transmural heterogeneity of ventricular repolarization under baseline and long QT conditions in the canine heart *in vivo*: torsades de pointes develops with halothane but not pentobarbital anesthesia. *J Cardiovasc Electrophysiol.* 2000;11:290–304.
4. Somberg J et al. Prolongation of QT interval and antiarrhythmic action of bepridil. *Am Heart J.* 1985;109:19–27.
5. Hill JA, Pepine CJ. Effects of bepridil on the resting electrocardiogram. *Int J Cardiol.* 1984;6:319–323.
6. Manouvrier J et al. Nine cases of torsade de pointes with bepridil administration. *Am Heart J.* 1986;111:1005–1007.
7. Cui G, Sen L, Sager P, et al. Effects of amiodarone, sematilide, and sotalol on QT dispersion. *Am J Cardiol.* 1994;74:896–900.
8. Torres V et al. QT prolongation and the antiarrhythmic efficacy of amiodarone. *J Am Coll Cardiol.* 1986;7:142–147.
9. Leroy G et al. F. Torsade de pointes during loading with amiodarone. *Eur Heart J.* 1987;8:541–543.
10. Burgess CD et al. The relationship between the QT interval and plasma amiodarone concentration in patients on long-term therapy. *Eur J Clin Pharmacol.* 1987;33:115–118.
11. Brown MA et al. Amiodarone-induced torsades de pointes. *Eur Heart J.* 1986;7:234–239.
12. Hohnloser SH, Klingenheben T, Singh BN. Amiodarone-associated proarrhythmic effects: a review with special reference to torsades de pointes tachycardia. *Ann Intern Med.* 1994;121:529–535.
13. Faggiano P et al. Torsades de pointes occurring early during oral amiodarone treatment. *Int J Cardiol.* 1996;55:205–208.
14. Nkomo VT, Shen WK. Amiodarone-induced long QT and polymorphic ventricular tachycardia. *Am J Emerg Med.* 2001;19:246–248.
15. Bergfeldt L, Schenck-Gustafsson K, Dahlqvist R. Comparative class I electrophysiologic and anticholinergic effects of disopyramide and its main metabolite (mono-*N*-dealkylated disopyramide) in healthy humans. *Cardiovasc Drugs Ther.* 1992;6:529–537.
16. Riccioni N, Castiglioni M, Bartolomei C. Disopyramide-induced QT prolongation and ventricular tachyarrhythmias. *Am Heart J.* 1983;105:870–871.
17. Kimura Y et al. Torsades de pointes in paced patients with sick sinus syndrome after disopyramide administration. *Jpn Heart J.* 1994;35:153–161.
18. Tzivoni D et al. Disopyramide-induced torsades de pointes. *Arch Intern Med.* 1981;141:946–947.

19. Boriani G et al. Repolarization changes in a double-blind crossover study of dofetilide versus sotalol in the treatment of ventricular tachycardia. *Pacing Clin Electrophysiol.* 2000;23:1935–1938.

20. Demolis JL et al. Influence of dofetilide on QT-interval duration and dispersion at various heart rates during exercise in humans. *Circulation.* 1996;94: 1592–1599.

21. Mazur A, Anderson ME, Bonney S, Roden DM. Pause-dependent polymorphic ventricular tachycardia during long-term treatment with dofetilide: a placebo-controlled, implantable cardioverter-defibrillator-based evaluation. *J Am Coll Cardiol..* 2001;37:1100–1105.

22. Stambler BS et al. Acute hemodynamic effects of intravenous ibutilide in patients with or without reduced left ventricular function. *Am J Cardiol.* 1997;80: 458–463.

23. Stevenson WG, Weiss J. Torsades de pointes due to *n*-acetylprocainamide. *Pacing Clin Electrophysiol.* 1985;8:528–531.

24. Piergies AA et al. Effect kinetics of *N*-acetylprocainamide-induced QT interval prolongation. *Clin Pharmacol Ther.* 1987;42:107–112.

25. Reiter MJ et al. Effects of quinidine versus procainamide on the QT interval. *Am J Cardiol.* 1986;58:512–516.

26. Fieldman A, Beebe RD, Sing Sum Chow M. The effect of quinidine sulfate on QRS duration and QT and systolic time intervals in man. *J Clin Pharmacol.* 1977;17:134–139.

27. Kopelman HA et al. Electrophysiologic effects of intravenous and oral sotalol for sustained ventricular tachycardia secondary to coronary artery disease. *Am J Cardiol.* 1988;61:1006–1011.

28. Kus T et al. Efficacy and electrophysiologic effects of oral sotalol in patients with sustained ventricular tachycardia caused by coronary artery disease. *Am Heart J.* 1992;123:82–89.

29. Kuhlkamp V et al. Efficacy and proarrhythmia with the use of d,l-sotalol for sustained ventricular tachyarrhythmias. *J Cardiovasc Pharmacol.* 1997;29: 373–381.

30. Cammu G et al. Two cases of torsades de pointes caused by sotalol therapy. *Resuscitation.* 1999;40:49–51.

31. Claghorn JL, Schroeder J, Goldstein BJ. Comparison of the electrocardiographic effect of dothiepin and amitriptyline. *J Clin Psychiatry.* 1984;45:291–293.

32. Dorsey ST, Biblo LA. Prolonged QT interval and torsades de pointes caused by the combination of fluconazole and amitriptyline. *Am J Emerg Med.* 2000;18:227–229.

33. Stern SL et al. 2-Hydroxydesipramine and desipramine plasma levels and electrocardiographic effects in depressed younger adults. *J Clin Psychopharmacol.* 1991;11:93–98.

34. Baker B et al. Electrocardiographic effects of fluoxetine and doxepin in patients with major depressive disorder. *J Clin Psychopharmacol.* 1997;17:15–21.

35. Alter P, Tontsch D, Grimm W. Doxepin-induced torsade de pointes tachycardia. *Ann Intern Med.* 2001;135:384–385.

36. Strasberg B et al. Doxepin induced torsade de pointes. *Pacing Clin Electrophysiol.* 1982;5:873–877.

37. Ohtani H, Odagiri Y, Sato H, et al. A comparative pharmacodynamic study of the arrhythmogenicity of antidepressants, fluvoxamine and imipramine, in guinea pigs. *Biol Pharm Bull.* 2001;24:550–554.

38. Monlun E et al. Prolonged QT interval with halofantrine. *Lancet.* 1993;341: 1541–1542.

39. Toivonen L et al. Provocation of ventricular tachycardia by antimalarial drug halofantrine in congenital long QT syndrome. *Clin Cardiol.* 1994;17:403–404.

40. Ohtani H et al. Comparative pharmacodynamic analysis of QT interval prolongation induced by the macrolides clarithromycin, roxithromycin, and azithromycin. *Chemotherapy.* 2000;44:2630–2637.

41. Lee KL et al. QT prolongation and torsades de pointes associated with clarithromycin. *Am J Med.* 1998;104:395–396.

42. Kamochi H et al. Clarithromycin associated with torsade de pointes. *Jpn Circ J.* 1999;63:421–422.

43. Mishra A, Friedman HS, Sinha AK. The effects of erythromycin on the electrocardiogram. *Chest..* 1999;115:983–986.

44. Rubart M et al. Electro-physiological mechanisms in a canine model of erythromycin-associated long QT syndrome. *Circulation.* 1993;88:1832–1844.

45. Tschida SJ et al. QTc-interval prolongation associated with slow intravenous erythromycin lactobionate infusions in critically ill patients: a prospective evaluation and review of the literature. *Pharmacotherapy.* 1996;16:663–674.

46. Katapadi K et al. A review of erythromycin-induced malignant tachyarrhythmia — torsade de pointes: a case report. *Angiology.* 1997;48:821–826.

47. Nattel S et al. Erythromycin-induced long QT syndrome: concordance with quinidine and underlying cellular electrophysiologic mechanism. *Am J Med.* 1990;89:235–238.

48. Oberg KC, Bauman JL. QT interval prolongation and torsades de pointes due to erythromycin lactobionate. *Pharmacotherapy.* 1995;15:687–692.

49. Wassmann S, Nickenig G, Bohm M. Long QT syndrome and torsade de pointes in a patient receiving fluconazole [letter]. *Ann Intern Med.* 1999;131:797.

50. Anderson ME et al. Potassium current antagonist properties and proarrhythmic consequences of quinolone antibiotics. *J Pharmacol Exp Ther.* 2001; 296:806–10.

51. Pohjola-Sintonen S et al. Itraconazole prevents terfenadine metabolism and increases risk of torsades de pointes ventricular tachycardia. *Eur J Clin Pharmacol..* 1993;45:191–193.

52. Zimmermann M et al. Torsades de pointes after treatment with terfenadine and ketoconazole. *Eur Heart J.* 1992;13:1002–1003.

53. Samaha FF. QTc interval prolongation and polymorphic ventricular tachycardia in association with levofloxacin [letter]. *Am J Med.* 1999;107:528–529.

54. White CM, Grant EM, Quintiliani R. Moxifloxacin does increase the corrected QT interval. *Clin Infect Dis.* 2001;33:1441–1442.

55. Demolis JL et al. Effect of a single oral dose of moxifloxacin (400 mg and 800 mg) on ventricular repolarization in healthy subjects. *Clin Pharmacol Ther.* 2000;68:658–666.

56. Wharton JM, Demopulos PA, Goldschlager N. Torsade de pointes during administration of pentamidine isethionate. *Am J Med.* 1987;83:571–576.

57. Bibler MR et al. Recurrent ventricular tachycardia due to pentamidine-induced cardiotoxicity. *Chest.* 1988;94:1303–1306.

58. Mitchell P et al. Torsades de pointes during intravenous pentamidine isethionate therapy. *Can Med Assoc J.* 1989;140:173–174.

59. Stein KM et al. Ventricular tachycardia and torsades de pointes complicating pentamidine therapy of *Pneumocystis carinii* pneumonia in the acquired immunodeficiency syndrome. *Am J Cardiol.* 1990;66:888–889.

60. Gonzalez A et al. Pentamidine-induced torsade de pointes. *Am Heart J.* 1991;122:1489–1492.

61. Mani S, Kocheril AG, Andriole VT. Case report: pentamidine and polymorphic ventricular tachycardia revisited. *Am J Med.* Sci 1993;305:236–240.

62. Eisenhauer MD et al. Incidence of cardiac arrhythmias during intravenous pentamidine therapy in HIV-infected patients. *Chest.* 1994;105:389–395.

63. Dupont H et al. Torsades de pointe probably related to sparfloxacin. *Eur J Clin Microbiol Infect Dis.* 1996;15:350–351.

64. Adamantidis MM et al. Sparfloxacin but not levofloxacin or ofloxacin prolongs cardiac repolarization in rabbit Purkinje fibers. *Fundam Clin Pharamcol.* 1998;12:70–76.

65. Weiner I et al. QT prolongation and paroxysmal ventricular tachycardia occurring during fever after trimethoprim-sulfamethoxazole administration. *Mt Sinai J Med.* 1981;48:53–55.

66. Lopez JA et al. QT prolongation and torsade de pointes after administration of trimethoprim-sulfamethoxazole. *Am J Cardiol.* 1987;59:376–377.

67. Little RE et al. Torsade de pointes and T-U wave alternans associated with arsenic poisoning. *Pacing Clin Electrophysiol.* 1990;13:164–170.

68. Beckman KJ et al. Arsenic-induced torsade de pointes. *Crit Care Med.* 1991;19:290–292.

69. Soignet SL et al. United States multicenter study of arsenic trioxide in relapsed acute promyelocytic leukemia. *J Clin Oncol.* 2001;19:3852–3860.

70. Unnikrishnan D et al. Torsades de pointes in 3 patients with leukemia treated with arsenic trioxide. *Blood.* 2001;97:1514–1516.

71. Ohnishi K et al. Prolongation of the QT interval and ventricular tachycardia in patients treated with arsenic trioxide for acute promyelocytic leukemia. *Ann Intern Med.* 2000;133:881–885.

72. Liu XK et al. The antiestrogen tamoxifen blocks the delayed rectifier potassium current, IKr, in rabbit ventricular myocytes. *J Pharmacol Exp Ther.* 1998;287:877–883.

73. Trump DL et al. High-dose oral tamoxifen, a potential multidrug-resistance-reversal agent: phase I trial in combination with vinblastine. *J Natl Cancer Inst.* 1992;84:1811–1816.

74. Hoehns JD et al. Torsades de pointes asociated with chlorpromazine: case report and review of associated ventricular arrhythmias. *Pharmacotherapy.* 2001;21:871–883.
75. Warner JP, Barnes TR, Henry JA. Electrocardiographic changes in patients receiving neuroleptic medication. *Acta Psychiatr Scand.* 1996;93:311–313.
76. DiSalvo TG, O'Gara PT. Torsade de pointes caused by high-dose intravenous haloperidol in cardiac patients. *Clin Cardiol.* 1995;18:285–290.
77. Hunt N, Stern TA. The association between intravenous haloperidol and torsades de pointes: three cases and a literature review. *Psychosomatics.* 1995;36:541–549.
78. Jackson T, Ditmanson L, Phibbs B. Torsade de pointes and low-dose oral haloperidol. *Arch Intern Med.* 1997;157:2013–2015.
79. Sharma ND et al. Torsades de pointes associated with intravenous haloperidol in critically ill patients. *Am J Cardiol.* 1998;81:238–240.
80. Lawrence KR, Nasraway SA. Conduction disturbances associated with administration of butyrophenone antipsychotics in the critically ill: a review of the literature. *Pharmacotherapy.* 1997;17:531–537.
81. Metzger E, Friedman R. Prolongation of the corrected QT and torsades de pointes cardiac arrhythmia associated with intravenous haloperidol in the medically ill. *J Clin Psychopharmacol.* 1993;13:128–132.
82. Hatta K et al. The association between intravenous haloperidol and prolonged QT interval. *J Clin Psychopharmacol.* 2001;21:257–261.
83. Dallaire S. Thioridazine (Mellaril) and mesoridazine (Serentil): prolongation of the QTc interval. *CMAJ.* 2001;164:91,95.
84. Krahenbuhl S et al. Case report: reversible QT prolongation with torsades de pointes in patients with pimozide intoxication. *Am J Med.* Sci 1995;309:315–316.
85. Gajwani P, Pozuelo L, Tesar GE. QT interval prolongation associated with quetiapine (Seroquel) overdose. *Psychosomatics.* 2000;41:63–65.
86. Beelen AP, Yeo KT, Lewis LD. Asymptomatic QTc prolongation associated with quetiapine fumarate overdose in a patient being treated with risperidone. *Hum Exp Toxicol.* 2001;20:215–219.
87. Hulisz DT et al. Complete heart block and torsae de pointes associated with thioridazine poisoning. *Pharmacotherapy.* 1994;14:239–245.
88. Buckley NA, Whyte IM, Dawson AH. Cardiotoxicity more common in thioridazine overdose than with other neuroleptics. *J Toxicol Clin Toxicol.* 1995;33:199–204.
89. Reilly JG et al. QTc-interval abnormalities and psychotropic drug therapy in psychiatric patients. *Lancet.* 2000;355:1048–1052.
90. Turgeon J et al. Block of IKs, the slow component of the delayed rectifier K^+ current, by the diuretic agent indapamide in guinea pig myocytes. *Circ Res.* 1994;75:879–886.
91. duBell WH et al. Effect of the immunosuppressant FK506 on excitation-contraction coupling and outward K+ currents in rat ventricular myocytes. *J Physiol.* 1997; 501: 509–516.
92. Johnson MC et al. QT prolongation and torsades de pointes after administration of FK506. *Transplantation.* 1992; 53: 929–930.

93. Hodak SP et al. QT prolongation and near fatal cardiac arrhythmia after intravenous tacrolimus administration. *Transplantation.* 1998; 66: 535–537.

94. Drolet B et al. Droperidol lengthens cardiac repolarization due to block of the rapid component of the delayed rectifier potassium current. *J Cardiovasc Electrophysiol.* 1999;10:1597–1604.

95. Lischke V et al. Droperidol causes a dose-dependent prolongation of the QT interval. *Anesth Analg.* 1994;79:983–986.

96. Harder S, Thurmann P. Clinically important drug interactions with anticoagulants: an update. *Clin Pharmacokinet.* 1996;30:416–444.

97. Wells PS et al. Interactions of Warfarin with drugs and food. *Ann Intern Med.* 1994;121:676–683.

98. Freedman MD, Olatidoye AG. Clinically significant drug interactions with the oral anticoagulants. *Drug Saf.* 1994;10:381–394.

99. Bristow MR et al. Early anthracycline cardiotoxicity. *Am J Med.* 1978;65: 828–832.

100. Weaver SK et al. A paucity of chronic electrocardiographic changes with adriamycin therapy. *J Electrocardiol.* 1978;11:233–238.

101. Bristow MR. Toxic cardiomyopathy due to doxorubicin. *Hosp Pract.* 1982;17:101–111.

102. Harrison DT, Sanders LA. Letter: pericarditis in a case of early daunorubicn cardiomyopathy. *Ann Intern Med.* 1976;85:339–341.

103. Bristow MR et al. Doxorubicin cardiomyopathy: evaluation by phonocardiography, endomyocardial biopsy, and cardiac catheterization. *Ann Intern Med.* 1978;88:168–175.

104. Von Hoff DD et al. Risk factors for doxorubicin-induced congestive heart failure. *Ann Intern Med.* 1979;91:710–717.

105. Von Hoff DD et al. Daunomycin-induced cardiotoxicity in children and adults: a review of 110 cases. *Am J Med.* 1977;62:200–208.

106. Villani F et al. Evaluation of cardiac toxicity of idarubicin (4-demethoxydaunorubicin). *Eur J Clin Oncol.* 1989;25:13–18.

107. Coleman RE et al. Mitoxantrone in advanced breast cancer: a phase II study with special attention to cardiotoxicity. *Eur J Cancer Clin Oncol.* 1984;6:771–776.

108. Henderson IC et al. Randomized clinical trial comparing mitoxantrone with doxorubicin in previously treated patients with breast cancer. *J Clin Oncol.* 1989;7:560–571.

109. Durkin WJ et al. Treatment of advanced lymphomas with bleomycin (NSC-125066). *Oncology.* 1976;33:140–145.

110. Ahmed M, Slayton RE. Report on drug-induced pericarditis. *Cancer Treat Rep.* 1980;64:353–355.

111. Corder MP, Flannery EF. Possible radiation pericarditis precipitated by actinomycin D. *Oncology.* 1974;30:81–84.

112. Klein K. Complications of testicular tumor therapy. *Int J Radiat Oncol Biol Phys.* 1977;2:1049–1051.

113. Buckner CD et al. High-dose cyclophosphamide therapy for malignant disease: toxicity, tumor response, and the effects of stored autologous marrow. *Cancer.* 1972;29:357–365.

114. Mills BA, Roberts RW. Cyclophosphamide-induced cardiomyopathy: a report of two cases and review of the English literature. *Cancer.* 1979;43:2223–2226.

115. Klein HO et al. High-dose ifosphamide and mesna as continuous infusion over five days: a phase I/II trial. *Cancer Treat Rev.* 1983;10(suppl A):167–173.

116. Einhorn LH. VP 16 plus ifosphamide plus cicplatin as salvage therapy in refractory testicular cancer. *Cancer Chemother Pharmacol.* 1986;18(suppl 2):S45–S50.

117. Talley RS et al. Clinical evaluation of toxic effects of cis-diamminedichloroplatinum (NSC-119875): phase I clinical study. *Cancer Chemother Rep.* 1973;57:465–471.

118. Hashimi LA, Khalyl MF, Salem PA. Supraventricular tachycardia: a probable complication of platinum treatment. *Oncology.* 1984;41:174–175.

119. Hartmann DW et al. Unanticipated side effects from treatment with high dose mechlorethamine in patients with malignant melanoma. *Cancer Treat Rep.* 1981;65:327–328.

120. Mancuso L et al. Cardiac toxicity of 5-fluorouracil: report of a case of spontaneous angina. *Tumori.* 1986;72:121–124.

121. Pottage A et al. Fluorouracil cardiotoxicity. *Br Med J.* 1978;6112:547.

122. Eskilsson J, Albertsson M, Mercke C. Adverse cardiac effects during induction chemotherapy treatment with cis-platin and 5-fluorouracil. *Radiother Oncol.* 1988;13:41–46.

123. Mandel EM, Lewinski U, Djaldetti M. Vincristine-induced myocardial infarction. *Cancer.* 1975;36:1979–1982.

124. Somers G et al. Myocardial infarction: a complication of vincristine treatment. *Lancet.* 1976;2:690.

13 Alternative Pharmacotherapy for Cardiovascular Diseases

Vitalina Rozenfeld

CONTENTS

0-58716-044-7/03/$0.00+$1.50

TABLE 13.1
Alternative Therapy for Management of Cardiovascular Diseases

Alternative Therapy	Indication(s)	Mechanism of Action/Active Ingredients	Dose	Side Effects	Drug Interactions
Artichoke (*Cynara scolymus* or *C. cardunculus*)	Hyperlipidemia	Contains cynarin and chlorogenic acid; cynaroside may inhibit HMG-CoA reductase	Typical dose 500 mg of dry leaf extract daily; 1800 mg per day has been used	Flatulence, increased bile flow, allergic reactions (especially if sensitive to Asteraceae/Compositae family, such as ragweed, chrysanthemums, marigolds, daisies)	
Bran (wheat: *Triticum aestrivum*, oat: *Avena sativa*, rice: *Oryza sativa*)	Hyperlipidemia, hypertension	Contains dietary fiber	Wheat bran: 20–35 g daily Oat bran: 3 g of soluble fiber (~38 g of oat bran or 75 g of dry oatmeal) daily Rice bran: 12–84 g rice bran or 4.8 g rice bran oil daily	Flatulence, bezoars, abdominal discomfort	May interfere with drug absorption; potentiation of hypoglycemic agents

Herb	Indications	Mechanism/Contains	Dosage	Adverse effects	Drug interactions
Butcher's broom (*Ruscus aculeatus*)	Circulatory disorders	Contains the steroid saponins ruscin and ruscoside	Raw extract equivalent to 7–11 mg total ruscogenin	Nausea, vomiting	
Coenzyme Q-10 (Ubiquinone)	Congestive heart failure, angina, hypertension	Antioxidant; a cofactor in ATP production; membrane stabilizer	Heart failure: 100 mg daily in 2–3 divided doses; Angina: 50 mg TID; Hypertension: 120 mg daily in 2 divided doses	Gastrointestinal disturbances: elevation of liver enzymes with doses >300 mg/day	Additive effects with antihypertensive agents; antagonism of Warfarin activity; reduction of CoQ-10 levels by beta-blockers, statins, and oral hypoglycemic agents
Fish oils	Hypertension, hyperlipidemia, coronary heart disease	Contain high amounts of omega-3 fatty acids eicosapentaenoic acid (EPA) and docosahexaenoic acid (DHA)	Fish oil: 1–4 g daily or EPA: 1–16 g daily; DHA: 1.8–2.8 g daily	Fishy taste, gastrointestinal symptoms, nosebleeds	Potentiation of antiplatelet/anticoagulant antihypertensive agents; enhanced effects of etretinate; increased risk of vitamin E deficiency with long-term use
Flaxseed (*Linum usitatissimum*)	Hyperlipidemia, reduction in platelet aggregation	Contains alpha-linolenic acid, which raises serum omega-3 polyunsaturated fatty acids level	Crushed seeds: 35–50 g daily; Oil: 15–30 ml daily	Diarrhea with doses >30 g per day	Potentiation of antiplatelet/anticoagulant agents

TABLE 13.1 (CONTINUED)
Alternative Therapy for Management of Cardiovascular Diseases

Alternative Therapy	Indication(s)	Mechanism of Action/Active Ingredients	Dose	Side Effects	Drug Interactions
Garlic (*Allium sativum*)	Hypelipidemia, hypertension, prevention of age-dependent vascular changes	Smooth muscle relaxation, HMG-CoA reductase inhibition, reduction in oxidative stress, antiplatelet effects	4 g fresh garlic (1 clove) or 600–1200 mg garlic powder/aged garlic extract daily	Gastrointestinal symptoms, changes to the intestinal flora, allergic reactions, garlic breath/odor	CYP3A4 inducer; also potentiation of antiplatelet/ anticoagulant/ hypoglycemic agents
Ginkgo biloba leaf extract (*Ginkgo biloba*)	Arterial occlusive disease, circulatory disorders	Improvement of blood flow and its rheological properties	120–160 mg native dry extract in 2 or 3 divided doses daily for at least 6 weeks	Gastrointestinal upsets, headaches, allergic skin reactions	Increases bleeding with antiplatelet/ anticoagulant agents; possibly inhibits CYP1A2 and CYP2D6; might affect CYP3A4
Guggul (*Commiphora mukul*)	Hyperlipidemia	Contains guggulsterone and gugulipid	100–500 mg guggulipid daily	Gastrointestinal upset, headache, hiccups	Reduced bioavailability of propranolol and diltiazem; interference with activity of thyroid agents (enhance effect of thyroid supplements)

Hawthorn leaf with flower (*Crataegus spp*)	Cardiac insufficiency, prevention of age-dependent vascular changes	Contains flavonoids and procyanidins, which have cardiotrophic properties	Powder: 200–500 mg tid; Tincture: 20 drops 2–3 times daily; Extract: 160–900 mg daily in 2-3 divided doses	Gastrointestinal upset, headache, palpitations, dizziness, agitation	Potentiate action of vasodilators, cardiac glycosides, antiarrhythmics, CNS depressants
Horse chestnut seed (*Aesculus hippocastanum*)	Venous insufficiency	Contains aescin with anti-exudative and has vascular-tightening properties; reduces the activity of lysosomal enzymes	100 mg aescin (250–312.5 mg extract) twice daily in delayed release form	Nausea, pruritis, gastric disturbances	Possible additive effects with anticoagulant/hypoglycemic agents
Hydroxymethylb utyrate (HMB)	Hyperlipidemia, hypertension	HMB is a by-product of leucine metabolism	3 g daily		
Indian snakeroot (*Rauvolfia serpentina*)	Hypertension, tachycardia	Contains reserpine alkaloids with sympatholytic activity (catecholamine reduction)	600 mg (6 mg total alkaloids content) daily	Stuffy nose, central nervous system depression, fatigue, reduction in libido	Digitalis glycosides (bradycardia), neurolpetics and barbiturates (potentiation), levodopa (reduced efficacy), sympathomimetics (initial exacerbation of hypertension)

TABLE 13.1 (CONTINUED)
Alternative Therapy for Management of Cardiovascular Diseases

Alternative Therapy	Indication(s)	Mechanism of Action/Active Ingredients	Dose	Side Effects	Drug Interactions
L-Carnitine	Congestive heart failure, myocardial infarction, hyperlipidemia, circulatory disorders	An essential cofactor for transport of long-chain fatty acids across membranes	2–4 g daily	Gastrointestinal distress, seizures	
Lily-of-the-valley herb (*Convallaria majalis*)	Cardiac insufficiency, cor pulmonale	Contains cardiac glycosides, which have positive inotropic and negative chronotropic effects	Average daily dosage: 0.6 g standardized lily-of-the-valley powder equivalent preparations; the effectiveness for the claimed application is not well documented	Nausea, vomiting, gastric disturbances, arrhythmias	Not to be used with digitalis glycosides or during hypercalcemia, hypokalemia, and conduction disturbances; increased toxicity with quinidine, calcium, diuretics, laxatives, and long-term glucocorticoid use
Lavender flower (*Lavandula angustifolia*)	Circulatory disorders	Contains linalyl acetate, camphor, *s*-ocimene, 1,8-cineol, and tannins	External use as bath additive: 20–100 g of drug for a 20-l bath	Contact dermatitis	Possible potentiation of CNS depressants

Motherwort (*Leonurus cardiaca*)	Tachycardia	Contains alkaloids (stachydrine), glycosides of bitter principles, and bufenolide	4.5 g daily	Diarrhea, stomach irritation, uterine bleeding, allergic reactions	Increased toxicity when used with cardiac glycosides
Onion (*Allium cepa*)	Atherosclerosis prevention	Inhibits platelet aggregation	Average daily dosage: 50 g of fresh onions or 20 g of dried drug equivalent preparations	Gastric disturbances	Potentiate effect of antiplatelet/anticoagulant/hypoglycemic agents
Olive oil (*Olea europaea*)	Prevent cardiovascular disease, hypertension, hyperlipidemia	Contains monounsaturated fatty acids (oleic, palmitic, linoleic)	Extra-virgin oil: 30–40 g daily in the diet	Biliary colic	Possible potentiation of hypoglycemic agents
Pheasant's eye herb (*Adonis vernalis*)	Cardiac insufficiency, circulatory disorders	Contains flavonoids and cardioactive glycosides	0.6 g of standardized adonis powder daily (not to exceed 3 g per day or 1 g as a single dose)	Nausea, vomiting, arrhythmias	Not to be used with digitalis glycosides or during hypercalcemia, hypokalemia, and conduction disturbances; increased toxicity with quinidine, calcium, diuretics, laxatives, and long-term glucocorticoid use

TABLE 13.1 (CONTINUED)
Alternative Therapy for Management of Cardiovascular Diseases

Alternative Therapy	Indication(s)	Mechanism of Action/Active Ingredients	Dose	Side Effects	Drug Interactions
Red yeast (*Monascus* spp); a component of Cholestin, which is being investigated by FDA as an unregulated drug	Hyperlipidemia	Contains mevinic acids (e.g., lovastatin), which inhibit HMG-CoA reductase	1200 mg two times daily with food	Abdominal discomfort, elevated liver enzymes	Lowering of CoQ-10 levels, enhanced effect of hepatotoxic agents, interaction with substances affecting CYP3A4 (e.g., grapefruit juice, St. John's wort)
Scotch broom herb (*Cytisus scoparius*)	Circulatory disorders	Contains alkaloids, primarily sparteine	Aqueous-ethanolic extracts equivalent to 1–1.5 g of drug daily	Dizziness, palpitations, headache	Due to the tyramine content, avoid using with MAOI; quinidine and haloperidol inhibit sparteine metabolism

Sitostanol	Hyperlipidemia	A saturated form of plant sterols that competitively inhibits dietary and biliary cholesterol absorption	800 mg to 4 g daily	Gastrointestinal upset	Reduced beta-carotene absorption; enhanced activity of lipid-lowering therapies
Soy (*Glycine max*)	Hyperlipidemia, hypertension, cardiovascular disease prevention	Contains isoflavones, which are hydrolyzed to phytoestrogens genistein and daidzein	Soy protein: 20–50 g daily	Gastrointestinal upset, allergic reactions	Possible competitive inhibition of estrogen replacement therapy effects; potential inhibition of thyroid hormone synthesis
Soy lecithin (*Glycine max*)	Hyperlipidemia	Contains (phosphatidyl)choline, phosphatidyl ethanolamine and phosphatidyl-inositol, which regenerate cell membranes and stop lipid peroxidation	Equivalent of 3.5 g (phosphatidyl)choline daily	Gastrointestinal upset	
Sweet clover (*Melilotus* spp)	Phlebitis, chronic venous insufficiency	Contains 5,6-benzo-pyrone (coumarin)	Equivalent of 3–30 mg coumarin daily	Headaches	Potentiate effects of anticoagulants

TABLE 13.1 (CONTINUED)
Alternative Therapy for Management of Cardiovascular Diseases

Alternative Therapy	Indication(s)	Mechanism of Action/Active Ingredients	Dose	Side Effects	Drug Interactions
Squill (*Urginea maritima*)	Cardiac insufficiency	Contains glycosides (scillaren A, proscillaridin A) and flavonoids; has positive inotropic and negative chronotropic effect	0.1–0.5 g of standardized sea onion daily	Gastrointestinal disturbances, arrhythmia	Efficacy/side effects augmented by quinidine, calcium, diuretics, laxatives, and extended glucocorticoid therapy

CYP3A4 = cytochrome P450 3A4; MAOI = monoamine oxidase inhibitors.

REFERENCES

Blumenthal. *The Complete German Commission E Monographs: Therapeutic Guide to Herbal Medicines*, American Botanical Council, 1998.

Jellin JM, Gregory P, Batz F, et al. Pharmacist's Letter/Prescriber's Letter/Natural Medicines Comprehensive Database. Stockton, CA: Therapeutic Research Faculty. http://www.naturaldatabase.com. Accessed July 2001.

AltMedDex® System. Micromedex Inc. Healthcare Series 1974-2001, Vol. 109 exp. 9/2001.

Robbers JE, Tyler VE. *Tyler's Herbs of Choice: The Therapeutic Use of Phytomedicinals*, 2nd ed., Haworth Press, 1999.

Index